CHANGE YOUR MIND, CHANGE YOUR BODY

CHANGE YOUR MIND, CHANGE YOUR BODY

Feeling Good About Your Body and Self After 40

Ann Kearney-Cooke, Ph.D.,

with Florence Isaacs

ATRIA BOOKS

NEW YORK   LONDON   TORONTO   SYDNEY

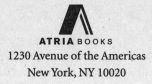

ATRIA BOOKS

1230 Avenue of the Americas
New York, NY 10020

Copyright © 2004 by Anne Kearney-Cooke, Ph.D., with Florence Isaacs

Library of Congress Cataloging-in-Publication Data is available

ISBN: 0-7434-3975-9

First Atria Books trade paperback edition June 2004

10 9 8 7 6 5 4 3 2 1

ATRIA BOOKS is a trademark of Simon & Schuster, Inc.

For information regarding special discounts for bulk purchases,
please contact Simon & Schuster Special Sales
at 1-800-456-6798 or business@simonandschuster.com

Manufactured in the United States of America

ACKNOWLEDGMENTS

—

Without the participation and help of significant people in my life, this book would not have been possible. My gratitude to them all.

I could not have researched and written *Change Your Mind, Change Your Body* without the love, understanding, and patience of my husband, Michael Cooke. I thank my adventurous, loving children, Kristin, Michael, Jenny, and Jonathan, who make me laugh and challenge me every step of the way.

I owe much to my parents, Gerry and the late Margaret Kearney, who believed in me and taught me to believe in myself. To my five siblings and their spouses: Jerry and Bonny, Billy and Patty, Regina and Timmy, Bobby and Kathy, and Peggy and Chuck, who reminded me to work hard and to never forget to have fun. To my nieces and nephews Erin, Megan, Sean, Christopher, Kegan, and Kelly; I am proud of each of you and look forward to many more reunions and parties at the beach.

To T. George Harris, who encouraged me throughout my career to keep up with the latest scientific research, to never stop asking the hard questions, and to be courageous and develop innovative, effective treatments for mental disorders.

To Marianne Lagota, M.D., founder and director of the Partnership for Gender Specific Medicine at Columbia University, whose brilliance and strength have inspired me and motivated me as they have all of the women she mentors and helps move forward in their careers.

To Susan Wooley, Ph.D., who early in my career encouraged and supported me to develop creative approaches to the treatment of body-image disturbance among women suffering with anorexia nervosa and bulimia nervosa.

Thanks to my colleagues and friends at the Academy of Eating Disorders, National Eating Disorder Organization, Eating Disorders Coalition, National Association of Anorexia and Associated Disorders, and Renfrew Center, with whom I have grown up professionally over the last twenty years. The members of these organizations are bright, talented, and dedicated to the prevention and treatment of eating disorders. In particular, thanks to Judith Rabinor, Ph.D.; Amy Baker Dennis, Ph.D.; Craig Johnson, Ph.D.; Michael Levine, Ph.D.; Melanie Katzman, Ph.D.—trusted colleagues and friends who I first met at the Columbus Conference on Eating Disorders twenty years ago. We have supported each other professionally and personally throughout the years.

Thanks to my outstanding colleagues at the Cincinnati Psychotherapy Institute; Sue McNeil, Ed.D.; Pam Owens, Ed.D.; Barbara Sween, Psy.D.; Terri Role Warren, Ph.D.; and Nicole Hemmert, R.D., a hardworking team focused on the treatment of eating disorders and body-image disturbance.

I want to thank Barbara Harris, editor-in-chief of *Shape* magazine, a woman of incredible integrity and insight, who taught me a holistic model of fitness and, along with Rebecca Gorrell, developed the Positive Body Project. Thanks to Kathy Soverow, M.A., a great visionary and leader, and Linda Shelton, M.A.; Gabriela Masali, M.A.; Kenya Masali, M.A.; and Lisa High, R.D. for the opportunity to work together on the amazing Shape Your Life Project. Thanks to the unrestricted educational grants from Secret antiperspirant brand of Procter and Gamble, I've had the opportunity to conduct research on adolescent girls and speak to underprivileged girls throughout the country with R & B singer

Mya and WNBA player Lisa Leslie about how to build physical, mental, and emotional strength in their lives.

Thanks to my incredible girlfriends, in particular the women of Mistymorn Lane and Indian Hill who are loyal friends, dedicated mothers, and effective in impacting the world around them.

Thanks to Linda Konner, my agent, who loved this project from the beginning, and Brenda Copeland, my editor, whose meticulous attention to all of the details and support throughout the book process has been invaluable. To Florence Isaacs, a terrific writer, who has taken my scientific and clinical style of writing and translated it into a language that readers can understand.

Finally I express my gratitude to the patients I have treated and the participants in the workshops I have led throughout the world. You have been my primary source of learning over the years. You have profoundly touched my mind, soul, and heart, and somewhere in this book I hope you can find what you have taught me, and the mark you have left.

CONTENTS

INTRODUCTION

—

When you look in the mirror, do any of the following statements come to mind:

"My dress is too tight. My waist is disappearing."

"I can't wear short sleeves anymore. My arms are too chunky."

"My makeup settles in the lines on my face."

"This haircut makes me look old. I looked better with long hair."

If you're over forty, most likely your answer is yes. Midlife is a time of change for you and your body. Some changes may be for the better, but others can leave you feeling anxious, ineffective, and out of control—especially when a youthful appearance is equated with sex appeal and is a ticket to approval and attention for women in our society.

We know from research that women's dissatisfaction with their bodies has skyrocketed since the 1960s, when worship of youth first came into vogue and ideals of beauty changed from the mature sensuous body of Elizabeth Taylor to the Twiggy look. It's fascinating that during the sixties and seventies, when women were gaining more economic and other power in the world, that a prepubescent girl became the ideal. Could the world not handle a mature, sensuous, and powerful woman? Creating an ideal that so few women could achieve keeps women in line—feeling bad about themselves. As women gained more freedom in the world, many felt imprisoned by this impossible ideal.

Literature specifically on female body image at midlife is scarce and inconclusive. Although most of it suggests that women over forty tend to be unhappy with their appearance, a few studies indicate the opposite. Clinical observation and case reports suggest that eating disorders are occurring with greater frequency in women over forty. Concerns about an aging appearance, including aging skin, can be associated with a drive for thinness and excessive dieting, factors that are key components in the development of eating disorders.[1]

Symptoms of eating disorders in midlife include: preoccupation with body image, use of over-the-counter or prescribed drugs to lose weight, exercise addiction, inability to make life transitions or to mourn significant losses, fear of aging, and unrealistic goals.[2]

In the workshops I conduct and in my private practice, I see many middle-aged women who don't like (or even hate) how they look—and the dissatisfaction affects virtually every aspect of their lives. Most do not meet the full diagnostic criteria for anorexia nervosa or bulimia nervosa, but have symptoms of a subclinical eating disorder such as restrictive dieting, exercise addiction, and obsession with their weight and shape. They come in to see me for other reasons, but their negative body image is what is holding them back. American culture has told them that they must have the bodies of twenty-year-olds to have value as women. Consequently, they long for and focus on an appearance that is impossible to achieve for all but a few. In pursuit of this elusive goal, they often engage in destructive behavior, such as yo-yo dieting. The investment takes so much time and energy (psychic and otherwise) that they have little left to put into anything else. Instead of using midlife as an opportunity to explore themselves and the world around them, they are imprisoned by an obsession with every piece of food they eat and with their weight.

When women fail to meet these impossible body-type standards, they feel bad about themselves. A forty-five- or fifty-year-old will tell me that she has no self-control, although she's a wonderful mother, or one of the best fund-raisers in the city, or renowned for her work in her field. Deep inside she doesn't experience her self-worth because her body isn't perfect. I've also seen how women project onto their bodies bad feelings about themselves or tension in their relationships, leading them to binge and/or become exercise addicts.

Nobody likes to see the signs of aging, and it's natural to wish that you didn't have crow's-feet, lines on your neck, or weight that just won't come off. We all struggle at times with negative feelings about our bodies, and there's more to be dissatisfied with after forty. But you don't have to dwell on inevitable changes or become depressed about them. You can focus on the possibilities you do have and get on with your life. You can move from thinking, "If I have a certain look I'll be sexy and attractive," to becoming a woman who honors the wisdom she has acquired over the years, knows who she is, and is sexy and attractive because of it.

The chapters ahead are not simply about accepting yourself, however. They are about sculpting yourself into a vibrant, adult woman and using the wisdom and experiences you've gained to shape a new vision of what you want your life to look like. Our society tells us that midlife, generally considered to be the years from forty to sixty-five, is a stage of decline. In reality, it is an opportunity for renewal and strength—a time to redefine who you are and what you want, and to set new goals.

I'm in midlife myself, and one of the things I love about being a baby boomer is being part of a group that questioned everything. We questioned as we marched in college, and we've continued to question and revise values we were taught about sex, politics, child rearing, women's roles, and virtually everything else. Yet we haven't questioned the issue of body image and a culture that tells us the ideal of beauty is a shape that is reed thin, rather than womanly, and that we're supposed to have that shape at forty, fifty, and beyond. Ours is the generation that attempted to overthrow institutions in the hope of building more meaningful ones. Yet we aspire to look like anorexic actresses and childlike models with vacant stares, many of whom have undergone cosmetic surgery, endure dangerous eating habits, and devote much of their lives to working out. We may have taken off the girdles our mothers wore, but we haven't discarded the girdle mentality.

We see women exercising tremendous power in business and government, running companies, and having babies at forty five. Yet we still let society dictate an ideal of beauty that is often impossible to achieve and sometimes unhealthy. And we beat ourselves up when we fall short of that ideal. In an era that heralds powerful women, a successful prosecutor is just as likely to spend lunch talking about how fat she is as about her latest case.

A BODY IMAGE REVOLUTION

Our bodies have been through a lot, and they're incredible. They menstruate every month, have babies, and then go through menopause. Yet rather than honor our bodies, we concentrate on what's wrong with them. All of us, no matter how attractive we are, want to lose weight. Isn't it past time to question this response—and rebel? Midlife is a chance to shift into another, more satisfying way of being, one that is centered not on a perfect appearance but on becoming more authentic and alive. It is an opportunity to embrace the many strengths you possess, expand your capabilities, and, in the process, live a more adventurous, pleasurable, and meaningful life.

Many women are afraid of change. Fear can freeze you into old patterns that don't work and hold you back. To get unstuck, you're going to need new skills. Part of my mission in this book is to provide them. Along the way, I will help you take a serious look at what you lose in midlife, what you can gain, and how to grow up and blossom. The fact is, you can become more fit, looking and feeling sexier than when you were younger, with new approaches to exercise. Fitness is a crucial goal because it maximizes your physical, emotional, and social abilities, which make you a more effective person. Building a resilient, strong body is as important as building a resilient, effective self in midlife. As your body grows stronger, you'll find that you also develop a stronger voice in the world and the power to handle what life throws your way.

The practical exercises and strategies in this book will help you deal with your fears of aging and turn them into tools for positive growth, emotional maturity, and increased spirituality. I will share creative strategies to help you overcome emotional eating and develop a healthy relationship with food. The stories of women from different ethnic groups will show you a different way to look at your own body. You will also learn how to help your daughter and other young women around you develop a healthy body image.

Part of your transformation will involve a whole new way of thinking about yourself and your appearance. You'll learn to look at the mistakes you've made as part of the fabric of life and use them as sources of information rather than reasons to punish yourself. You will search within to develop your own beauty ideal. This is important because body dissatisfaction derives from the practice of judging yourself as deviating from the cultural standards of attractiveness. Remember, grown-up appeal, sexual and otherwise, is about attitude and energy, strong bodies, and openness to new possibilities. These traits are ageless and timeless, and others are drawn to them.

You won't make the shift to loving your body and yourself overnight. But by consistently and repeatedly practicing the techniques that follow, you will find that you gradually spend more of your time accepting your body and less time criticizing it. When you do feel bad about your appearance, you'll learn ways to restore your newfound body acceptance faster. A little bit of change each day eventually leads to a marked improvement in body image.

Middle age is the prime of your life—a time to renegotiate your relationship with your body, your self, and those around you. Read on to discover the power in your body and in your ability to move ahead in new directions.

HOW DO YOU FEEL ABOUT YOUR BODY NOW?

Body image is the mental picture you have of your body, including thoughts and feelings about your physical self. We all have everyday issues with body image, which are often magnified by the physical changes that take place at midlife. This quiz will help clarify your own feelings and attitudes about your appearance, and identify behaviors that can be damaging.

Circle the answer that applies.

1. I feel generally satisfied with my body.
> a. True
> b. Somewhat true
> c. False

2. I have at least some attractive physical attributes.
> a. True
> b. Somewhat true
> c. False

3. I feel self-conscious about my body.
> a. Rarely or never

       b. Sometimes

       c. Usually

4. I usually compare my body to the bodies of other women

       a. my own age.

       b. somewhat younger.

       c. under thirty.

5. When someone compliments me on the way I look, I usually feel

       a. flattered.

       b. skeptical.

       c. self-conscious.

6. I worry about the effect of aging on my looks.

       a. Never

       b. Occasionally

       d. Most of the time

7. I exercise

       a. at least three times a week.

       b. a few times a month.

       c. rarely or never.

8. I have taken diet pills, fasted, or followed an extremely low-calorie diet.

       a. Rarely or never

       b. At least once in the past year

       c. Several times in the last year

9. Compared to five years ago, I feel that I look

       a. better.

    b. the same.

    c. worse.

CHECK YOUR ANSWERS

1. Your answer to this question is important because unhappiness about appearance erodes self-esteem and can lead to unhealthy behaviors. Recently I pulled out and examined the responses of 282 midlife women, aged forty to sixty, to a 1997 survey I conducted of *Shape* magazine readers. I found that 58 percent were dissatisfied with their appearance, a very high level of discontent, and one that can contribute to low self-esteem.

2. Too often we focus on our flaws and pay little or no attention to our appearance strengths, which we all have. In responses to a 1999 *Shape* magazine survey I conducted, 86.4 percent of midlife women were satisfied with their hair; 86 percent with their facial attractiveness; 61.7 percent with their arms; 72.7 percent with their chest/breasts; 61.8 percent with their legs; and 62.8 percent with their muscle tone. Name three of your own appearance strengths. Be sure to include assets such as graceful hands and beautiful eyes.

3. Self-consciousness is evidence of dissatisfaction with the body. In a 1997 *Shape* magazine survey, 85 percent of midlife respondents acknowledged some level of self-consciousness about their appearance. Self-consciousness often leads to behaviors like "hiding the body" and feelings of shame and withdrawal from others. Make a list of the times you are overly self-conscious about your body. Think of different ways you can talk to yourself during these times and move through space in a more confident manner.

4. If you contrast yourself with cover girls twenty or thirty years younger, you are setting yourself up to feel bad. Re-

search[3] suggests that comparing yourself to your peers may help maintain your self-esteem and your satisfaction with life in spite of age-related losses.

5. Inability to respond to, accept, or feel comfortable with compliments is a common sign of a negative body image. This robs you of the pleasure of feeling good about your body. It also robs the giver of warm feelings. A compliment is actually a gift.

6. A study of 125 women aged fifty to sixty-five and 125 women sixty-six and older[4] found a direct relationship between fear of aging and body dissatisfaction, increased binge eating, and an inability to listen to body signals, such as hunger. Research indicates that a concern with aging can be associated with a drive for thinness and excessive dieting, which may precipitate the development of eating disorders, osteoporosis, and stress fractures, due to nutritional deficiencies.[5]

7. Midlife *Shape* magazine readers with a positive body image were more likely to exercise—and to exercise more often—than those who were dissatisfied with their bodies. Regular exercise makes a difference in how you look by firming and toning your body, and helping to control weight. Exercise also builds confidence—and confidence is an essential factor in sex appeal.

8. *Shape* magazine research found that unhealthy weight control efforts are more likely to be used by women who are dissatisfied with their bodies than by satisfied women. Other research[6] found a direct correlation between dissatisfaction with the body and women who believe weight loss is associated with youthful looks.

9. There is a double standard of aging for men and women in America. Men are perceived as more attractive and appealing to women as they age, but women tend to view

themselves as less attractive and less desirable as they age. Have you bought into this? Remember that you are a grown woman, not a young girl. You can challenge this double standard. I know and have treated women in midlife who, at the completion of therapy, actually feel more attractive and desirable after forty because of choices they make each day in the way they treat their bodies. For example, research on 144 men and women aged twenty to eighty found that getting older was associated with greater body satisfaction for women who exercised.[7] Midlife can actually be a season of your life when you feel better—not worse—about your body.

INTERPRETING YOUR SCORE

You *can* learn a whole new way of looking at your body and yourself. But first you need insight into what's going on. If you circled mostly *a*s, you seem to feel generally positive about your body. Keep it up. If you circled mostly *c*'s, you owe it to yourself to make changes. Negative feelings and attitudes can interfere with your life and erode self-esteem. It's important to explore what gets in the way of accepting your body. If you circled a relatively equal mix of *a*'s, *b*'s, and *c*'s, your body image could be improved. Can you see areas and attitudes that need work?

PART ONE

Is Your Body Image Realistic?

1

DO YOU HAVE A PROBLEM WITH YOUR AGE?

The Grand Canyon has been and continues to be formed by cataclysmic events, as well as millions of momentary changes. Still the whole is ever present, the changing yet undiminished. I ask myself, "Why are we afraid of dramatic or devastating change in our life, in ourselves? Is it possible to recast what we perceive to be negative, as something beautiful, something sculpting our lives, our psyches, our souls. Aren't we, like the canyon, made new again and again, yet always intimately whole?"

—Kathleen Jo Ryan,
Writing Down the River

You are a woman of forty, or forty-five, or fifty-one. The next half of your life lies ahead of you. Do you want to spend it fighting your body, or fixing what you can, accepting what you can't, and embracing the power within you? A lot of dissatisfaction with the body in midlife is really about aging and failure to come to terms with it. Sometimes you use your body as a screen upon which you project negative feelings about other aspects of your life.

The fact is, your body is changing and will continue to do so. Instead of fearing change, you can use it to grow stronger, more fulfilled, and happier with yourself and your life. Accomplishing that, however, requires acknowledging and dealing with the real anxieties all of us experience about aging.

HOW DO YOU FEEL ABOUT GETTING OLDER?

Our culture makes it difficult to accept the process of getting older. It encourages an endless adolescence. Although we used to see beauty in voluptuous, strong women like Sophia Loren and Elizabeth Taylor, the ideals today are teen idols. Youth dictates the trends in fashion and TV.

How do you experience your own aging? Does getting older mean moving from being a girl to being an old lady? A patient of mine told me, "I look old. I feel old." She's fifty-one, and she's bought into the myths of our culture—that the glorified qualities of adolescence equal beauty, that getting older means being unattractive, asexual, and less valued.

In fact, there is a great big middle ground between being a girl and an old lady. It is being a woman—someone who knows who she is, what she wants, and how to go after it. A woman is wiser, more confident, and sexier in her way. A woman takes responsibility for her needs and takes credit for her strengths. She honors the knowledge that she's gained and a history of perseverance and effort in the obstacles she's overcome. That rich history didn't exist when you were twenty-something. When you give voice to that part of yourself, you move through the world in a way that is very attractive and alluring.

I see the transformation in my own patients. Initially, they come to me blaming their unhappiness on their thighs or faces. But they discover it goes far deeper than that, and that they have the power to effect change in their bodies and themselves. The same power exists in you. You can feel helpless when you confront the first signs of aging, but watching and despairing are not your only choices. There's another way to go. You can learn to change some of your attitudes and develop new skills as you move ahead in your life. But first you need to deal with unfinished business that can get in the way.

LOOKING AT LOSSES

The reality is, as we get older, we face very real losses in our lives, such as loss of parents or loss of a goal or dream. Because these losses are rarely acknowledged as such, they often linger in the shadows, becoming roadblocks to positive change. But if you look at them openly, you don't have to fight them. You can put the energy of ignoring your losses elsewhere. Let's examine these losses of midlife and see how they may affect you.

Loss of Youthful Appearance

As you get older, you may notice that fewer men turn around when you walk down the street. You are referred to as "ma'am" and treated in a different manner. The signs of aging may be most painful for those of us who have defined ourselves by our looks and sexuality. In a way, age is the great equalizer—the former prom queen has more to lose than the wallflower.

How do you experience the signs of losing your youthful appearance? Nobody wants to get older, of course, but do you generally accept it and get on with your life? Or do you tend to obsess about your face, flabby arms, and the rest of your body? If you do obsess over aging, it stops you from living and enjoying your life to the fullest. Negative feelings about your body affect your moods, your eating habits, your sex life, and your relationships. That's why it's important to develop many sources of self-esteem, such as close relationships with others or involvement in meaningful work, whether paid or unpaid—not just appearance.

Loss of Menstrual Cycle

The upside of losing your menstrual cycle is the opportunity for a freer, more spontaneous sex life. You no longer have to worry about pregnancy. But other issues arise.

Some women mourn the loss of fertility. A door has permanently closed. They've lost the option to have children, or to bear more children, and they may have regrets.

For example, I've seen some lesbian women in midlife who look back and recall that twenty-five years ago it was not acceptable for a lesbian to bear a child. Yet today they see younger lesbian women feeling free to do so. They wish they had had the opportunity to become parents.

Some women miss the rhythms of the menstrual cycle. I see participants in my groups who have irregular periods during perimenopause, the time preceding menopause when levels of the hormones estrogen and progesterone decline. They are not sure from month to month whether or not they will have a period, and the uncertainty leads them to feel out of control. Sharing with the group personal accounts of what they are experiencing helps them accept menopausal changes more easily. A woman will say, "I don't have a period at all for three months and then suddenly I get this incredibly heavy period." Others in the group respond by sharing similar experiences and ideas on how to deal with this, and they all wind up laughing about their unpredictable lives.

In addition, some women in my groups had children in their twenties, while others waited until their thirties or even forties. Those who became mothers later often feel excited but tired. For many women who had children earlier, the question is, What is your role once you can no longer bear children? The answer is they can move from focusing on their role as parent to greater focus on their own autonomy and self-care. This transition can be difficult, because social norms have established a woman's role as caring for others—and cultural messages requiring women to put others' needs first must be challenged. Often women see the move to taking better care of themselves as becoming selfish.

I urge these women to say to themselves, "I'm not being selfish—I'm building a self. And that's the best investment I can make in maintaining my quality of life into old age."

There are other concerns, as well. If you don't dread the loss of your menstrual cycle, then you probably, like most women, dread the changes associated with menopause, such as hot flashes and loss of energy. You may also worry that because of menopausal changes you won't feel very sexual, you'll have vaginal dryness, and the changes will affect your sexual performance. Lubricants, hormone replacement therapy (if you are a candidate), and other options can help. Your health and sexuality, in fact, can reach their peak in midlife if you can learn to celebrate your body and yourself.

Empty Nest

When children leave home, the structure that has surrounded them disappears. This affects all moms to some degree but is particularly difficult for full-time homemakers. When your kids move on to college or other choices, there's something exciting about it—it frees up your time and allows you to address your own needs more immediately. But even positive changes involve loss. If your identity has been based largely on being a mother, you do feel the pain of that changing role.

A few years ago, Theresa,* a forty-eight-year-old patient of mine, vacationed in Italy for ten days with her husband. She immediately experienced the loss of separation from her three children. She felt a bit overwhelmed at being in a strange country and found herself clinging to her husband at times.

---

*Names and identifying details in personal stories have been changed to protect privacy.

"The worst thing was the day I got home," she told me. "One of my kids really missed me, but the others did great. My mother, who watched them, said there wasn't even that much work. My husband said I should feel so proud, that it means the kids are independent. They can operate without us. But what I feel is sadness because my whole identity is what I do for them. I feel that I have no worth because it doesn't matter if I'm here or not."

Although this is an extreme example, most mothers can identify with some of these feelings. When you can let yourself feel the pain of loss fully and grieve for it, you can eventually let go of the sadness. You can transform it into energy to pursue something else. For Theresa, the trip was the beginning of her grieving and beginning to accept that there's a point at which your children don't need you in the same way. Your identity and good feelings are going to have to come from something different.

Women who worked full-time while raising their children have additional issues to face as kids leave. Some regret spending too much time building a career rather than being with their children when they were young. I see many women who feel the pain of opportunity lost, yet who also see chances to forge a new relationship with their children. They make sure that they are involved in their kids' adult lives. They never miss college weekends. They go to help out for two weeks when a daughter or daughter-in-law has a baby. And they are loving, attentive grandparents.

Some women, however, channel their empty nest sadness into eating. They head straight for the refrigerator, and the pounds go on. Other women move in the opposite direction, thinking, "Okay, now that the kids are gone, my energy is going into looking great." It's a good thing to take better care of yourself, but for some women it becomes an addiction. Their mental energy revolves around diets, face-lifts, and how many hours they can exercise a day. This attitude disempowers women because there's a limit to the amount you can do with your body. Even if you do two hours of aerobics a day or lose five more pounds, you've still lost that piece of your identity or that way to structure your life if you haven't replaced it with something else.

Do you find yourself overeating—or, just as bad, dwelling on diets, liposuction, or plastic surgery? Then it's time to ask, Will overeating or obsessing about losing weight or erasing the lines on my neck really make me happy? Or is this a distraction, a way of not looking at other issues in my life?

Loss of Parents

The changing relationship with your parents represents another loss at midlife. As you get older, they grow frail. In a role reversal, they may not only be unable to lend a helping hand to you but they may also need you to help care for them.

Vangie, a forty-six-year-old psychologist, experienced this role reversal when her mother was diagnosed with cancer. Since Vangie had children later in life, her two sons were young. She loved that her parents truly enjoyed the boys, babysat them on Saturday mornings, and attended all their athletic events. Within a year of her mother's diagnosis, however, everything changed. Instead of Vangie's parents providing help, enthusiasm, and comfort, they were depressed and needed her support. Her father had to deal with the effects of caring for his desperately ill wife. Her mother never felt well, and was less attentive to, or interested in, Vangie and the children.

This was an unexpected loss for Vangie, but one that led her to learn to reach outside the family to others. She began to attend a cancer support group for the families of patients. Here, she was able to talk about her fears about her mother dying and express a spectrum of other feelings, such as anger and sadness. Sharing honestly with others in similar situations helped her grieve her loss and get through this difficult time.

Loss of Peers

When your own peers are diagnosed with terminal illness, you begin to feel how fast time is moving and how soon life can end. It's a sobering realization that can paralyze you—or lead you to reassess what you want in life, set priorities, and act on them. For example, Rachel, a patient of mine, was shocked when Alan, her best friend's husband, died at forty-five. A policeman who ran daily and rock climbed, Alan was one of the fittest men on the police force. He had grown up with Rachel and her friend. How could he die so young?

As Rachel and her widowed friend grieved together, they pulled out photograph albums and looked at snapshots of Alan and themselves as teenagers. "I hadn't seen these pictures in many years, and I was surprised to see the good shape I was in. I had always felt overweight then. I thought I was never thin enough," Rachel told me.

"And here I am twenty-five years later, still worrying about how I look, when Alan has died. His life is over. I don't have time for this anymore." Rachel was alive, and she realized that she wanted help in therapy to change her focus on appearance.

Changes in Your Health

At midlife, you may feel a vulnerability about your own health for the first time. One woman who grows her own herbs explained, "I love to garden, but I notice that I can't do it for long stretches anymore. My joints stiffen much sooner." Suddenly she is aware that her health isn't what it used to be.

Serious conditions such as diabetes, arthritis, and heart disease begin to appear in midlife, and one in every fifteen women will develop breast cancer between thirty-five and fifty-five. Such realities can motivate you to adopt a healthier lifestyle, or they can lead you into feelings of hopelessness and depression. Which way do you want to go? Many women in my groups feel that through exercise, taking vitamins, and staying out of the sun, they can do something to counter the effects of aging. They are making active efforts to prevent disease.

Loss of Goals and Dreams

Many of my midlife patients come to me because they just got divorced, or they're in pain about the choices they've made that are irreversible. Some losses involve old goals and dreams that have been forgotten or compromised over the years. A woman may realize that she'll never be the ballerina she had once hoped to be. Some may never have a happy marriage with two kids in the suburbs. Spouses may be blamed bitterly for lost dreams. To get past such losses, women must not only mourn the way they've spent their adult years but also honor the road taken. You can't be who you are without all the choices you've made, both the good and the bad. You need to appreciate how much you've grown as a result of your choices.

You may think, "I never pursued my career. I raised my children instead, and now that they are away at school, I have nothing." But part of who you are at this moment is all the things you learned as you raised your children. You can transform that learning into something else now.

And don't forget what a powerful effect you've had on your children's lives. You may lament, "Why did I have to work so hard when my kids were little?" You owe it to yourself to honor that choice, and honor yourself as a role model to your kids. They got to see a woman being effective in the world. They saw how you handled challenges, and how you recovered when your work life tipped out of balance.

MOVING AHEAD

Whatever midlife losses apply to you, bring them out into the light. Allow yourself to feel the pain. Only then can you truly move on.

Different losses contribute to the experience of loss of a former younger self, which often makes women feel sad. It's a period of transition, but the exciting prospect is that you can transform yourself into a wiser new you.

Let me tell you about how a patient of mine is dealing with her losses. At age forty-eight, Jane has experienced both a breast cancer scare and the effects of an empty nest as her daughter, the eldest of three children, has gone off to college this year. Her daughter is struggling with being away at school and comes home every weekend. Jane struggles with it, too. She feels the loss of her daughter profoundly. The two of them used to watch TV together at night. They used to shop together. They did the dishes together and talked.

Jane has two other children still at home, but they are boys. Her daughter is her confidante and close friend. Jane's husband, although a good and loyal man, eats dinner after work and heads for the computer. Jane, who is thirty pounds overweight, fills the void with food and TV. Unconsciously, eating is a way to avoid grieving for the loss of her daughter at home. Jane dislikes her body shape and weight, and describes herself as looking frumpy.

In Jane's case, I helped her talk through the pain of "losing" her daughter, and helped her grieve. I also pointed out that she was reinforcing her daughter's difficult adjustment to college because she felt so lost and lonely herself. Jane's daughter felt guilty about leaving her mother. Because her daughter had spent so much of her time meeting Jane's needs, she had developed few outside relationships. She was afraid to be on her own.

Jane needed to get out of the house and try something different. I asked her, "What one thing would you like to do that is not at all like you?" She answered, "I'd love to go to San Francisco by myself to visit an old friend." For the first time in her life, Jane focused on herself and taking care of her own needs. She decided to take that trip. She bought the airline tickets and flew on a plane alone for the first time. She stayed with her friend, who has young children and was happy to have Jane go off on her own during the day. Jane would leave in the morning and explore the city, returning at 6 P.M. to spend the evening with her friend.

"Here I was in San Francisco and I found my way around. I felt so proud of myself," Jane told me. "I walked everywhere. I talked to people. I went to art museums. Nobody in my family would have been interested, but I loved it.

"This is the first time in my life I didn't have to plan my schedule around everyone else's. I woke up, ate what I wanted, when I wanted. If I wanted to go to a restaurant, I did. If I wanted to just have a pretzel for lunch from a stand, I did that." Interestingly, her trip marked the first time her daughter didn't come home for the weekend—and it's leading to other changes. Jane has joined a book club and now talks of signing up for a yoga class. Who knows? She may even pry her husband away from his computer, which marital therapy was unable to do. She's certainly becoming a more interesting woman to talk to.

Jane has found an adventurous part of herself, which gives her daughter permission to move on and find an adventurous part of herself. Her daughter has made new friends at school and is building a social life.

Simultaneously, Jane is overeating less. She originally came to see me about her weight, but the real issue wasn't her body—it was being stuck in an old pattern. She couldn't break out of that pattern until she grieved for her loss, experienced the emptiness, and opened herself up to possibilities.

Jane bought the idea that you always put others first, and she never thought of herself in a role other than caretaker for her children. Yet all of her children will leave home eventually. It was scary for her to confront the question, Who am I then? But conflict and instability are part of change. The answer is to embrace them.

OUTSIDE THE CAGE

If you ask people what they regret, it's usually actions they haven't taken: risks like pursuing educational opportunities, having children (if they did not), or having more children. Taking a risk and trying something different is what I call moving outside the cage. What is this cage I'm talking about? I learned about the cage from a story my father told me when I was in college, struggling with choosing a major and other personal decisions. It changed my life then and continues to guide me today.

> *There was once a community that was so proud of its zoo that it raised money to acquire a polar bear. In preparation, the zoo staff began to build an elaborate natural habitat to accommodate the bear and make it feel at home. People were very excited about it. But the polar bear arrived earlier than expected, over a month before the habitat was ready. To keep the bear healthy and comfortable in the meantime, a temporary cage was constructed at the edge of the habitat. For thirty-five days, the bear paced around the cage in the same kind of circling pattern.*
>
> *On the day that the habitat was ready, the community held a gala ribbon-cutting ceremony. The entire town showed up, happy and proud. As the cage was removed, everyone waited expectantly for the bear to walk into the spacious new habitat, exploring the terrain and all the water holes that had been provided. Instead, the polar bear continued to pace around in a circle as if still enclosed by the cage. The old limits, although invisible, remained.*

My father was trying to tell me that I was still stuck in an old vision of myself, with old boundaries and expectations of others. It was time for me to get out of the cage. I often tell this story because, like the bear, many of us remain inside the cage at midlife, restricted by old limits that no longer apply. It's scary to venture out of the cage, because you're accustomed to it, even though it prevents growth. But when you find the courage to do so, it's going to lead you to an exciting new life.

Although change is frightening and difficult, not changing is sometimes even harder. We forget how much energy is expended on staying stuck and often, how much suffering accompanies it. It takes effort to avoid a major issue, to procrastinate over a decision, and that effort often involves numbing behaviors like overeating, overworking, or drinking alcohol. Is staying in place easier if you have to drink two glasses of wine every night to medicate yourself? Is it scarier to open up and get closer to others than to bury fears of intimacy by working all the time?

Moving outside the cage can be especially important if you are employed. Working women often face both personal and career-related crises in midlife. The challenge may be how to slow down and deal with too much structure in your life, rather than too little. Take Phyllis, a partner in a Chicago law firm. Married for twenty-five years, she is the mother of three. She's achieved the success she's always wanted, but she's also deeply depressed. She feels tired. In the past, she always liked her appearance, but now she's having trouble living with a body and face that looks older. The reality is, she is a very attractive fifty-year-old.

Phyllis has had Botox injections, which temporarily reduce wrinkles, and has considered plastic surgery. She feels she is getting fat. "I diet, then I slack off, and I'm heavier than ever. I never thought I'd obsess about these things," she explains, "yet I look in the mirror and I'm flabby. I'm not very sexual anymore, and I don't feel good about myself."

Superficially, women think it's the spreading waist or age spots that are at the root of their dissatisfaction, but once they look deeply, they learn that other issues lie beneath. At this time of life, there are not only losses. You're also outgrowing activities and attitudes.

Phyllis feels she's on a treadmill working fourteen-hour days and traveling too much. She told me, "I keep saying to myself, 'Once I get to this spot, I won't be working so many hours.' Or 'Once I get to that, I won't have to do the community work.' But I've realized I'm fifty and my life hasn't changed. I'm not happy."

She also feels envious of her son, who is away at college on the West Coast. She muses, "What would it be like to be nineteen again and out in California, walking on the beach, falling in love, and talking about politics? I'm tired of going to dinner parties with my friends. We're all middle-aged, and it's the same old same old. And maybe you're right. It's not the wrinkles on my face or the weight in the middle of my body that's the problem. It's that I don't feel like I've been living for a long time. I feel like a robot."

For Phyllis, the big problem isn't losing her youthful appearance. She needs to deal with her dissatisfaction with her frantic work schedule and extra time she spends on community work to help attract new business. Obsessing over her appearance is a way of not looking at what's going on in her life.

I am working with Phyllis to redefine her role in her firm. We're talking about her slowing down and using the wisdom she's gained as a lawyer. She doesn't have to be on every board. Instead of being out on business three nights a week, she can reduce her rainmaking role and move further into work she enjoys: management, mentoring, and training younger associates. It may be time to shake up her social life: invite new friends for dinner parties, take a dance class with her husband, etc.

TUNE IN TO YOUR FEELINGS

To help midlife women recognize what's going on internally and begin to move outside the cage, I ask them to do this exercise. Try it for yourself:

Write the word "aging" in the middle of a piece of paper. Then close your eyes and jot down any other words that come to mind. No censoring or editing allowed. See what comes out. Write the words all over the page. Then take all these words and use them to write a letter to someone or to write a short story. You can use each word as many times as you want, but you must use all the words.

ROSE'S STORY

When I asked my client, Rose, a forty-five-year-old human resources director in Miami, to try this exercise, she came up with the following words:

old	wrinkled	aches and pains
worn	gray hair	memory fading
wise	maturing	illness
saggy	spirited	unafraid
mentor	inevitable	like a fine wine
getting better	getting worse	like a good cheese
getting on with it		

This is the story Rose wrote:

> *She had seen it all, done it all, and now she looked back at all*
> *the people and events that had shaped her life. Yes, while ma-*
> *turing, she had acquired the typical aches and pains of an old*
> *woman, but the deep wrinkles, gray hair, and saggy muscles*
> *had not drained her spirited personality. At times she felt that*
> *like a fine wine or a good cheese, she had gotten better with*
> *age. She had grown wise and been unafraid of the future as*
> *uncertain as it might seem. Lately, chronic illness had slowed*
> *her and she felt worn out, like she was getting worse. The un-*
> *speakable, inevitable lay ahead. She was afraid to be alone. Yet*
> *her friends were still close and a great comfort to her. They*
> *often reminisced about the neighborhood parties, the dinners*
> *at their favorite restaurants, and the band. With memory fad-*
> *ing, she still felt she could be a mentor to others, leaving a*
> *legacy to her children and grandchildren. She was getting on*
> *with it, getting on with her life.*

Rose, the mother of two teenagers, wrote this story imagining herself at the end of life. She illustrates her resiliency in handling ups and downs, and she has had her share of heartache. In the last two years, her husband left her, and both her parents succumbed to cancer. She's made it through the divorce and her parents' deaths. She's been able to grieve those losses.

Although disturbed by the physical changes of aging, she's confident they won't stand in her way. She's able to hang on to good memories of friends and family. But her story reveals that she needs to work through her anxieties about being alone for the first time in her life and her fears (unfounded so far) that her family history will cause illness to strike her next.

CARLA'S STORY

This exercise can pinpoint areas of dissatisfaction, often turning up issues about values, and relationships with husband, children, friends, and work. For example, Carla, a forty-six-year-old accountant, maintained a low-profile practice that enabled her to put family duties first. She liked that arrangement, but she was very dissatisfied with the same old routine in her relationship with her husband. She felt stuck and projected that onto her body, dwelling on being overweight.

A part of her story read:

She was married to a handsome prince who loved her, but it was a marriage steeped in tradition. History would dictate that the expectations of her job as princess included remaining loyal to the prince. She saw this as her duty, and she always fulfilled her obligations. She knew that if she left her role as a princess, she would never forgive herself for breaking the prince's heart. Still, the routines and habits they had fallen into left her sad and tired. Once she raised her two sons, she thought she would be free, but instead she felt trapped. Yet others around her seemed content. She wondered if something was wrong with her.

Carla was beginning to question unwritten rules about the roles she and her husband held. They operated in an emotionally disengaged marriage, which avoided conflict but resulted in boredom. When people ignore conflicts between them, the problems don't disappear. Women are often afraid to discuss with their husbands what's really going on. They fear opening a Pandora's box that will split the marriage. Ironically, not opening the box is a far greater threat to the relationship. The effect is deadening.

As shown in her words, Carla felt her only options were to stay in her marriage and suffer, or leave and feel guilty. I helped her focus on a third option: She and her husband could grow and change together. Her complaints of boredom and lack of intimacy with her husband were actually opportunities to set goals instead of getting depressed and eating. When you feel down and dissatisfied, overdosing on chocolates isn't what will remedy these feelings. You need other sources of pleasure. These can involve new, yet simple, changes in routines, such as breaking out of your vacation rut and going someplace different, expanding your social circle, and/or following new interests.

Carla found the courage to discuss her dissatisfaction with her husband, which led him to start talking about his discontents. This conversation opened a whole new dialogue between them.

So far, Carla and her husband have decided to shake up their vacation pattern of two weeks in Maine every August. They're taking a Caribbean cruise instead. They also plan to get active at the art museum and meet some new people. They're entering an exciting new phase of married life. It's full of risks, yes, but also rewards.

After you've written your story, show it to a trusted friend, someone in your age group who can empathize, understand, and discuss it with you. This can help you talk through your dissatisfactions and the pain of losses, whatever they are. It can help you examine questions such as, How do I want to live now that my children are growing up? What will make me happy? How will I relate to men sexually? How can I honor the wisdom I've gained through my years of experience? When you embrace these questions and combine them with new perspectives, midlife becomes an exciting process of transformation.

Part of this process includes celebrating the power of your body as experienced through menarche, pregnancy, menopause, and sexuality through the life span. Do you remember how it felt to be sixteen? No, you're not sixteen anymore, but you can have a strong body and feel your physical power through weight training and attention to fitness. You can find creative ways to look great, such as using a personal shopper (available free in many department stores) who can find the most flattering clothes and colors for you.

You can also define your success by self improvement instead of triumph over others. Good feelings don't have to come from "I exercise more than my neighbor next door." They can come from goals that are important to you and which you are setting and meeting. Channel competitive feelings, which we all have at times, into being the best you can be, whatever the endeavor—which is different from being better than someone else. Stop comparing yourself, because that leads to body hatred.

I'm going to challenge you to break out of your cage and become the writer of your own story, rather than someone acting out a role in a drama someone else has created. In the pages ahead, you'll find tools to help you take what you know and honor it instead of feeling bitter that you didn't take another route.

You have thirty or forty years ahead of you. Are you going to spend them worrying about the last ten pounds? Or are you going to grow up, learn from your failures instead of being demoralized by them, and use your considerable strengths?

2

ORIGINS OF YOUR BODY IMAGE

Every mother contains her daughter in herself and every daughter her mother, and every woman extends backwards into her mother and forwards into her daughter.

—C. G. Jung,
The Archetypes and the Collective Unconscious

At a resort in Mexico, a forty-five-year-old woman in shorts and a T-shirt sits at the edge the pool watching her children. Once a lifeguard who couldn't keep out of the water, she hasn't worn a bathing suit in years. Other women, many heavier than she, wear bathing suits. "My stomach sticks out and my thighs are too big to wear a bathing suit," she explains.

It's ninety-nine degrees in the shade as an attractive brunette sips latte at a café with a friend. Swathed in a black, long-sleeved dress with a high neck, she looks like an Italian widow. "My arms are heavy. I never wear anything sleeveless," she observes. "I also have lines on my neck."

A man asks his wife to dance at a family wedding. Although she loves the music and the dancing looks like fun, she grimaces and points him to a female relative. "Ask her," she suggests. "You know what a terrible dancer I am."

These women—all in midlife—weren't born hiding their bodies or feeling self-conscious about the way they move. There are other reasons why they, like many of us, have trouble tolerating a less-than-perfect appearance. Part of the explanation lies in how body image unfolds from childhood. To trace the origins of negative body image, I've created a model of body image development. It is based on my twenty years of clinical observations, my overview of scientific research in the field, and hundreds of hours in my workshops and other events throughout the country spent listening to women who have everyday issues with body image.

A negative body image involves multiple factors, such as *dissatisfaction with body size,* wherein your true body size differs from your concept of an ideal body; *dissatisfaction with shape,* or viewing yourself as fat and unattractive; and *body distortion,* in which your body, and your perception of your body's true size or appearance, are not the same. When you experience body distortion, you experience the body as fatter or thinner than it actually is, or a particular characteristic, such as hips or a nose, is viewed as bigger or uglier than it is, despite evidence to the contrary.

In creating my model, I found that certain psychological and sociological processes play a role in the development of negative body image. The four processes that follow will help you understand why some people feel terribly unhappy with their body, while others (who may even be less attractive) feel content. They will also shed light on what's getting in the way of your own body acceptance.

INTERNALIZATION

This is a progressive process in which we internalize—that is, take in and make part of our beliefs—the way our body has been talked about and treated by our peers, our parents, and others around us throughout our development. These are actual, re-peated experiences that children and significant adults share, which become a working model for the child's body image. A healthy body image is likely to develop when you are regularly treated with respect, both physically and emotionally.

Mary, a fifty-two-year-old college professor who sought ther-apy for depression, had a very different experience. A major source of her depression was dissatisfaction with her body. She constantly put down her appearance, never feeling attractive enough. "Being around critical people leaves its scars," she told me. "Both my parents were very critical of their children. They tended to focus on everything negative about us. As a result, I concentrate on what's wrong with me. Instead of saying, 'I have a nice figure,' I say, 'I have a big butt.' It's very hard to break this process. It's as if the critical words of your parents are being burned in your heart and mind. It's like being branded for life."

To illustrate the power of this branding, I ask women in my workshops, "How many of you have had a physical injury, such as a sprained ankle, or a broken arm or foot? Raise your hands." Many will do so. I follow up with, "If that broken bone or sprained ankle still hurts today, keep your hand raised." Only one or two will usually do so. Then I'll ask, "How many of you can re-member something that was said to you that was painful? The words could concern your body or anything else." Many raise their hands. I continue, "And how many of you still feel hurt or bad about it?" Several women keep their hands up.

The old saying "Sticks and stones will break my bones but words will never harm me" is not true. The impact of words remains with you—and they can harm you. A woman in one of my workshops recalled, "My father did not pay much attention to me. I always felt that he didn't think I was pretty. My mom was extremely control-ling, making critical remarks about my weight and shape. Both parents focused on the negative, and that's what I do."

To help patients work through these negative experiences, I encourage them to reconstruct the key relationships and events they've internalized that have left them feeling bad about their bodies. These can include a lack of loving touch, teasing, or abusive experiences.

Florence, my coauthor, for example, always felt that she was clumsy. She traced that feeling back to age five, when she took tap dancing and ballet lessons at a local dance studio, along with other little girls in her neighborhood. She'd practice at home in the large kitchen, which was the center of family activity. As she rehearsed the new steps she'd learned that week, she occasionally stumbled. Her mother would laughingly say, "You're a klutz."

If you repeatedly hear that from your parent and absorb that assessment as part of your body image, you're probably not going to be as creative and free when you move, and especially while you're dancing, as someone who hasn't been criticized. You're probably going to be self-conscious and indeed look clumsy.

As a five-year-old practicing your dance lessons, you expect your mother to mirror you, to feel as excited as you are about what you're doing and about the new skills you're learning. You're trying to enjoy how effective and beautiful your body is and you want her to say, "Keep it up." Instead, you're told, "You've done something wrong. Don't do that."

The criticism becomes part of your body image. That's going to affect the way you move through space, and therefore how others respond to you. People react differently to someone who glides gracefully down the street than to someone who moves awkwardly. It is not surprising that Florence avoided social dancing in her teen years, largely limiting herself to the fox trot. She considered herself a terrible dancer. Now the mother of two grown sons, she still does.

Another issue is involved, as well. Children are vulnerable when they go into the kitchen or living room and show off their dance steps, or their new backhand or serve on the tennis court. If criticized rather than encouraged most of the time, that response can become a template for the youngster. The lesson may be, "When I'm the center of attention, I'd better be careful. Something bad could happen. I could be criticized or ridiculed." This can have a ripple effect through the years, contributing to fear of success in an adult career and reluctance to take credit for accomplishments. The criticism also affects how you talk about yourself. One reason so many women feel comfortable putting down their own bodies is that it will make them more acceptable to other women. Say, "I look like a Sherman tank," and you're one of the girls. But if you add a positive statement such as, "I love how strong my body has grown," others often don't know how to respond. Later on in this book, you're going to learn how to teach yourself and other people to talk about your body so that the words do not harm your self-esteem.

Research shows that parents have increasingly negative perceptions and attitudes regarding their children's physical appearance as youngsters get older.[1] A daughter's beauty is very important to mothers. Girls hear this message loud and clear from Mom and internalize it. It's interesting that one study of girls with facial deformities and their mothers found that the youngsters were very dissatisfied with their bodies in general, not just their faces.[2] The authors suggested that these mothers placed great value on beauty and appearance.

Other researchers have looked at the relationship between parents' evaluation of their children's weight and the adolescent's own perception. They found that parental assessment of the weight was a more powerful predictor of how children perceived their own weight than their demographic characteristics or the physician's determination.[3]

DADDY'S ROLE

Fathers can have a tremendous impact on their daughters' body image, as well. As a daughter enters adolescence, she turns to the attention of her father and searches for his support for her changing body. The father's reaction to her physical maturation plays a role in shaping her feelings about becoming a woman. The quality of the emotional engagement between the father and daughter may become a template for future relationships with men. His views on the ideal body for women, his general attitudes toward women's bodies, and his comments about his daughter's maturity affect her body image in a positive or negative way.

My patient Irene, who obsessed over her weight, grew up in a working-class family where weekends centered around watching football on TV. After she left for college, she, like so many students, gained ten pounds in her freshman year. She remembers coming home one weekend and joining her father and brothers in the finished basement to watch a game. As she reached for a candy bar, her father warned her, "You know you're not going to be able to eat that kind of food anymore. You're getting heavy."

Until that moment, she had simply accepted her weight gain. All of her friends at college had gained weight too. They weren't getting much exercise at school and pigged out on junk food while studying. She didn't consider the extra pounds a big deal. But her father's comment, which also set off a barrage of criticism from her brothers, suddenly focused her on how she looked. "When the cheerleaders came on during halftime, and my brothers talked about how beautiful they were, I started comparing my body to their bodies and thinking, 'I really have gotten fat.' "

That day was the beginning of Irene's obsession with weight. Although she came into treatment twenty-eight years later, she could still recall her father's words. "I look at pictures of myself back then, and I certainly wasn't fat," she observes. "Yet my brothers said, 'Oh boy, you're really getting big hips,' which instantly made me self-conscious. I went on my first diet the next day." That began a cycle of yo-yo dieting, which became a way of life for her. She felt that her father was displeased with her, and she was someone who tried to please adults. "I remember that incident even today when I'm in the mood to eat a chocolate bar," she says. "I think, 'Oh no, you can't have candy.' " Oddly enough, she now realizes that her father was overweight. "Why was he allowed to have candy and popcorn while watching football and I was not?" she asks.

When I talk to women in my practice about body dissatisfaction, I find that it usually started in adolescence. I ask them to bring in pictures of themselves as teenagers. When they do, it's not uncommon for them to remark, "I'm surprised at how thin I looked. I really was in good shape, although my memory of the time was that I was always overweight."

Fathers don't necessarily have to be critical, however; some of them simply withdraw. Another patient, fifty-two, recalls, "My father was deathly afraid of my sexuality and developing body. I often felt being feminine was bad." In such cases, the daughter feels that all of a sudden she's gotten her period and she's starting to mature—and Dad has pulled away from her.

The woman above internalized her father's fear as her own fear that she would be abandoned—or that something bad would happen if she became comfortable with being a woman. I see this often in patients suffering from eating disorders.

It's important for fathers to relate in a different way toward their daughters in puberty. Girls will lament, "I used to wrestle with my father on the floor and now he's stopped doing that." It's appropriate that fathers cease that kind of activity, but daughters don't always understand that. They only know that Dad seems to have backed off. Sometimes, however, the father overdoes it. A daughter will complain, "My dad used to play tennis with me and then we'd go out to lunch and hang out together on Saturday. He doesn't do that anymore." The big issue is that Dad withdraws from physical contact. It's almost as if some fathers are so nervous about even the appearance of inappropriate touching that they just refrain from touching their daughters at all. The daughter interprets his response as, "It's bad for me to become sexy and mature." She associates it with a kind of loss.

How did your father treat you as an adolescent? Did he celebrate your emerging womanliness—or did he withdraw, or comment negatively about it, making you more self-conscious of the changes in your body? What was his concept of an ideal woman? Did he like voluptuous females or deride them as fat? Did he admire athletic women or call them lesbians? Such attitudes color your own feelings about your body and whether you think that you measure up.

PHYSICAL AND SEXUAL ABUSE

The effects of physical or sexual abuse can also be internalized. When a woman is sexually abused, the feeling is that her body is dirty, shameful, and something to be hidden. A study[4] on sexual abuse, which I coauthored with Diann M. Ackard, Ph.D., involved a sample of 1,664 female respondents to a survey in *Shape* magazine. Half the women said they had been sexually abused; the other half said they had not been abused.

We found that those who had been sexually abused had a more negative body image than women who were not. (We matched them on age and body mass index (BMI) to rule out these factors, which tend to affect body image: In general, the younger you are, the more unhappy you are with your body; the more overweight you are, the more dissatisfied you feel.) Abused women were more dissatisfied and self-conscious about their bodies. Most said that they felt very ashamed of their bodies. They were more uncomfortable about undressing in front of a partner and about having sex with the lights on.

They were less satisfied with themselves and their relationships, as well. This is not surprising, since sexual abuse destroys trust, which is the foundation of meaningful relationships.

There can be other consequences of sexual abuse, as well, such as identity confusion and eating disorders. The drive for thinness, which is idolized in our society, may reduce feelings of body hatred. If a woman blames her body for everything wrong with her, she may feel she can fix the problem by eliminating fat and making that body disappear. For someone sexually abused, trying to control the body can also be a way to try to regain control of herself. At the opposite end of the spectrum, women who are very frightened of others' attention on their body overeat because becoming fat wards people off.

Physically abused women report effects similar to those experienced by victims of sexual abuse, such as body image dissatisfaction.

Medical experiences that involve alteration of the body can be negatively internalized as well. A body changing medical procedure can negatively impact the body image of adults. For instance, breast cancer treatment may significantly change the body. Many women go through a long physical and mental healing process to restore a positive body image after their treatment. Some children who suffer with disorders such as inflammatory bowel disease (IBD) may experience multiple surgeries, or treatment with steroids, which causes them to gain weight at different points. Because the body changes a great deal, these youngsters may not have a chance to develop a stable image of the body. They don't feel normal.

We internalize the way our body is talked about and touched or not touched, and we also internalize feelings in reaction to traumatic experiences. In many ways our bodies contain our life stories. In the next section you will have an opportunity to learn more about your body image history.

TRACE YOUR HISTORY WITH A TIMELINE

What negative messages about your body did you internalize from significant people or experiences in your life? To reconstruct key relationships and events—and question unconscious assumptions and behaviors that may be damaging to you—it's helpful to keep a timeline of your body image history with the chart that follows. Close your eyes, relax, and begin to see pictures of how your body looked at various ages, starting at age five. Rather than rely solely on memory, you can either go back and actually look at pictures of yourself at that age, or you can ask people who knew you then to tell you what your body looked like and how it moved.

TIMELINE			
Age	Description of Body	Description of Meals, Snacks	What Was Going On in Family
5			
10			
15			
20			
30			
Present Age			

Say to yourself, "Now I'm five years old." Imagine how your body looks at this age. How does it move through space? Does your body seem to enjoy its freedom? Describe your shape and weight. What does your body say to the world? Describe typical meals and snacks, so that you can recognize the stage at which you started to have problems with food. It often helps to see the connection between how you feel about your body and how you eat. What was going on in your family and community? To confirm your memories, talk to relatives and family friends who knew you then.

Many women began to experience body image problems during transitions—their parents divorced, or the family moved from one state to another, or a brother was diagnosed with leukemia. When a transition is taking place, a child feels a loss of control and tries to exert control over the one thing she is solely responsible for, her body.

Do the same thing at ten. Has anything changed about the way you move now or the way you eat compared to age five? Continue the same way at ten, fifteen, twenty, thirty, and then at your present age. It helps you to see that the way you relate to your body is often similar to the way you relate to people and to food. For example, one woman noted that whenever a separation occurred, such as going away to college (or her son's departure for college), she wound up using food to soothe her anxiety.

CORINNE'S TIMELINE

I asked Corinne, fifty-four, a client of Chinese descent, to do a timeline, which provided some fascinating information. A petite, elegant dynamo who managed an upscale boutique, Corinne hated the way she looked. "I'm never going to get through midlife," she assured me. "When I see myself in the mirror every day, I'm obsessed with my wrinkles and sags. I watch older customers coming into the store and it makes me sick that I'm going to look like them at some point."

Corinne's timeline revealed that her family moved when she was eight years old. They left an ethnic neighborhood full of other Asian families for one that was more expensive, fashionable, and mostly Caucasian. In the new school, Corinne was one of only three Asian students.

Through the timeline, she realized that her body image problems started after that move. At age five, she saw herself skipping rope, running, rolling on the grass, and otherwise actively engaged in the environment. At age ten, however, the timeline indicated that she felt self-conscious about her looks. Some of her schoolmates made fun of her "Chinky eyes" and other Asian characteristics. She lived in this neighborhood until age fourteen. By then the experience had made a profoundly negative impact on her body image. She no longer felt good about her appearance. Corinne's dissatisfaction with her body didn't start with midlife wrinkles, it was rooted in childhood.

As Corinne worked on the timeline, she also uncovered another issue involving her parents, who owned a successful travel agency. When they made their upwardly mobile move, both her mother and father started working longer hours to pay for the more expensive house. Because they came home exhausted and stressed out, they argued more. These memories helped Corinne realize how powerless she felt to handle the difficult home atmosphere. When she complained to her parents that they were hardly at home anymore, they retorted, "If you want to live in a nice house, you have to see less of us." She would reply, "I don't care about living this way. I want my parents back." But they were committed to their upscale lifestyle.

It was then, Corinne realized, that she began to obsess about her weight.

Try the timeline yourself. See what you uncover about the origins of your body image.

PROJECTION

Projection is the second process that leads to a distorted body image. Your body can become a screen on which you project negative feelings you have about yourself. Or projection can occur when you feel overwhelmed by anxiety or other feelings that are difficult to handle. Because the body is perceived as perhaps the one thing you can control, changing it through weight loss or cosmetic surgery can offer the illusion of mastery. In reality, you gain anything but mastery, because the underlying issues—your feelings—are never addressed.

That's what happened in Corinne's case. In adolescence, as she dwelled on her appearance, her subconscious thinking went something like: "I may not be able to control my home life, but I can make a perfect body." Her need to look perfect resurfaced in midlife. She really struggled with her body then because, although she knew she was attractive and at a normal weight, she felt stuck in her marriage. In her childhood, she had felt at the mercy of those she'd depended on—her parents. As an adult, she felt at the mercy of her husband, whom she depended on now.

This left her feeling powerless and out of control. She thought the lines and wrinkles on her face were bothering her most, but the real problem was that she became obsessed with her looks whenever she felt impotent. Instead of owning the frightening feeling and dealing with it, she focused on her appearance.

We all project onto our bodies to some degree, but people often project more during transitions. I believe that midlife leaves women vulnerable to projection because it involves multiple transitions: Children are leaving or gone; we're coping with issues of whether to start or slow down a career; and menopause or perimenopause is beginning. Often there is also a transition in the relationship with a spouse or partner. All of these transitions play a role in a woman's focus on the imperfections of her body.

For example, a patient will tell me that her marriage is in trouble and that she can't seem to get what she needs from the relationship. "When I was busy raising the kids I think I ignored this," she'll say, "but now that the kids are older I'm aware of it. My husband doesn't seem happy either. I'm in turmoil because I can't do anything about it. I find myself constantly exercising and sometimes not eating." It's almost as if her inability to revive the relationship leads her to think, "If I can just get my body back in shape, I can revive my marriage."

Projection can also occur in response to other factors. For example, a woman may go to a PTA meeting where conflict rages over fund-raising approaches. People argue loudly, and she feels inadequate dealing with the dissension. It makes her feel out of control. This is a common situation, because many women do not tolerate conflict well. A whole body of research shows that women grow through relationships. The feeling of connection is important to us, and there's a sense that the only way to keep the connection is to eliminate discord. When conflict occurs, we fear that something bad will happen.

At the PTA meeting, instead of recognizing, "I feel out of control when people disagree," the woman projects, "My body is out of control—my thighs are enormous." She finds herself obsessively checking the fat content of everything she eats. She can't control the fact that it's hard for her to tolerate conflict, but she can control how much fat she eats today.

When you feel fat or old, are you distracting yourself from personal struggles or feelings that are difficult to handle? I always tell women, "Make believe you're coming home from work. All of a sudden you look down at yourself and say, 'My thighs are huge. They're disgusting.' You need to remember that you have the same thighs all day long. The fact that you're focusing on them right now may have some other meaning, because the size of your thighs hasn't changed since breakfast. Is there something else going on?"

A device I use called a decoding sheet can help you notice when and why you project so that you can do something about it. For one week, keep track of all the feelings about your body that you experience. Each day jot down the time, situation, and the particular feeling in the appropriate columns. The goal is to recognize the times that you are criticizing your body and see them as a signal to stop, identify the feeling, and try to understand what's really going on.

In order to decode your feelings you need to ask, "What am I trying to distract myself from at this moment?" Your entry might look something like, "At 9 P.M., when I climbed into bed, why did I all of a sudden feel the rolls on my stomach and get disgusted with them? Am I distracting myself from the fact that my husband is always watching TV in the den and never in bed with me? And is my unhappiness about that the true issue here?" Once you identify the real issue that's causing your feelings, you can develop an action plan. Answer the question, What do I need to do about this? You might write, "Improve my relationship with my husband" or "Learn to tolerate conflict." It is important that you realize that conflict is part of life. It's going to exist in situations where people are honest and share their ideas. It's normal and natural for people to disagree.

DECODING SHEET					
Day	Time	Situation	Feeling	Decode: This Thought Distracts Me From	Action Plan
Monday					
Tuesday					
Wednesday					
Thursday					
Friday					
Saturday					
Sunday					

ANOREXIA NERVOSA

I've found that women suffering from anorexia nervosa project onto their bodies when they are unable to handle difficult emotions and conflicts in their lives. I've found that when they experience an appetite for food and people, this is frightening to them because people have disappointed them in the past. When that appetite appears, they begin to feel out of control and project the feeling onto the body. The story of Evelyn, forty-three, illustrates the phenomenon. After struggling with anorexia nervosa for years, she entered group therapy.

Group members used the decoding sheet to keep track of the times each day that they felt negatively about their bodies—and of the people involved and the events that occurred at such times. Evelyn had decided to spend mealtimes with others, since she tended to eat more when she was with people. On the sheet, she reported that she had planned to join her sister and brother-in-law for dinner on a Friday night. The couple, who had been out golfing, had gotten delayed and had not come to pick up Evelyn for dinner on time. Evelyn had begun to feel physical hunger. However, eating a snack would not have helped her. The problem was that hunger of any kind frightened her, and she'd tried to avoid feeling it. In addition, she'd yearned to be out with her sister, rather than alone at home. Needing people left her feeling vulnerable because people had been so toxic in her life. She'd projected this overwhelming feeling onto her body. She reported having felt fat, flabby, and afraid that she was gaining too much weight. In response, she'd gotten on her treadmill and begun to discount her yearnings to be with her sister. As she'd sweated and burned calories, she'd begun to feel better. She'd convinced herself that the problem had not been that *she'd* felt out of control but that her body had been out of control. Jumping on an exercise machine had been a way to regain it.

Through our work in the group, Evelyn began to see that whenever she felt hungry for people or food, she felt out of control, which led to a distortion of her body image. The distortion switched her focus from the situation to changing her body—which actually played an important role in maintaining her eating disorder. Because most of Evelyn's time was spent changing the body, she remained unequipped to cope with the real issues. She did not develop skills to handle overwhelming feelings or interpersonal deficits, such as problems with intimacy, which caused profound feelings of inadequacy.

Although most women's struggles with body image aren't as severe as Evelyn's, the result is similar. If you work out on an exercise machine to avoid conflict, you still aren't equipped to handle the next PTA meeting. As more discord occurs there, you still feel uncomfortable, because the underlying issue is being ignored: You need to learn to tolerate conflict and see it as part of the fabric of life.

You're probably wondering, "How can I feel whole and okay even when people are mad or disagree with me—or when I'm experiencing an emotion that is difficult for me to handle? What do I do at such times?"

First, know that the situation or feeling will not go on forever. It can also be helpful to write in your journal. Just allow your thoughts to flow as you write and see where they lead you. Talking the issue over with a friend, as well as brainstorming strategies to deal with your discomfort, can help too.

There's an addictive component to projection and the distorted thinking that follows it. For example, alcoholics will say, "If I drink two martinis, I'll feel more relaxed at the party." But martinis will not relax them, so they have two more. Similarly, losing weight does not eliminate feelings of shame or increase the capacity for intimacy, which leads the person to feel that she has to lose more weight. This addictive element is apparent in the stories of body dysmorphic patients who hate their bodies. They constantly try to change imperfections, usually through plastic surgery, but they're never satisfied. They reconstruct their nose, but that's not enough to make them feel better, so they redo their eyelids. But that isn't enough either, and they have to try another procedure.

Is the drive for a perfect body distracting you? Ask yourself, "Is it a way to fill in emptiness or isolation which I feel in my life?"

IDENTIFICATION

My mother has always been critical of her own body and more critical of mine. She is always talking about how fat she is. She told me that when she was growing up, her best friend was gorgeous but she was plain. She got stuck with the guys her friend didn't want. She told me how she couldn't go to her first few job interviews after college because she felt too fat. Like my mom, even though people tell me I'm attractive, I feel ugly and fat. I always wanted to be one of those girls who stood out and was really pretty, but I feel invisible most of the time when I'm with people.

Do these words resonate with you? We all know that a strong bond exists between mothers and daughters. We're likely to mimic our mother's values and lifestyles as we mature, and identify with many of her attitudes and behaviors. You may not be aware, however, of how much you identify with how your mom felt about her own body. What others said about her appearance can affect you, as well.

Part of the reason for this identification is the fact that Mom is usually in charge of physical appearance expectations in the household. And research suggests that women who are critical of their own bodies tend to be more critical of how their daughters look.[5] Daughters whose mothers berated their own bodies had worse body images themselves than others did, and they tended to use more extreme weight loss measures. Did you hear comments from your mother such as, "I never look good. I'm getting too fat. These wrinkles are destroying my face"? If so, do you think such statements affected your body image?

The goal isn't to blame mothers here. They get blamed enough. But mothers often talk about their bodies in a negative way because they're feeling negative, and that does affect their daughters' body image.

You can turn this knowledge into an opportunity for you and your mother to talk to each other and heal. It's important to encourage each other to engage in healthy behaviors. You will find detailed advice on how to change damaging habits and how to be a role model and forge a new path with your own daughter in chapter 10.

IDENTIFY YOUR MOTHER'S BODY IMAGE ATTITUDES

How can you recognize your mother's feelings about her body? Try this exercise. Close your eyes and imagine you're a child of seven, eight, or nine, watching your mother dress to go out to a social event. Does she take a shower or bath? What's the expression on her face as she washes and dries herself, touching different parts of her body? Does she look pleased—or not? As she looks in the mirror while dressing and applying makeup, do you hear remarks such as, "This sure is a great color on me." Or, "Boy, I still have those great legs." Or does she make disparaging remarks?

Then talk to your mother about what you saw and heard to discover whether your impressions were real or distorted. When the two of you dialogue in this way, you can learn a great deal about each other. You realize how your mother talks about and treats her body, and how she moves in space. You also see how much you identify with her and the role that identification plays in your body image.

CULTURE

TV, movies, and billboards treat women as objects and say that our power lies in a perfect body. These messages can reinforce the damaging effects of internalization, projection, and identification. Do you buy into them? Many women in this country do, developing unrealistic standards of beauty. Then they apply those standards to themselves. For instance, we know that by age six, children have internalized the ideals of the culture—that thin is in and fat is bad.

Since the arrival of Twiggy in the 1960s, the ideals of beauty have stabilized at 13 percent to 19 percent below expected weight. These numbers are disturbing because body weight below 15 percent of expected weight is one of the diagnostic criteria for anorexia nervosa.[6] Researchers examined archival data of reported height and weight measurements of Miss America Pageant contestants from 1979 to 1988 and reported bust, waist, and hip measurements of *Playboy* centerfolds over a span of ten years. They found that 69 percent of the *Playboy* centerfolds and 60 percent of Miss America contestants weighed 15 percent or more below the expected weight for their age and height.[7] Leading ladies in some of the top TV series look anorexic, and stories in the tabloids document their struggles with that disorder.

How has the culture of thinness affected your feelings about your body? In a Swiss study of midlife and older women, 71 percent wanted to be thinner even though 73 percent of them were of normal weight.[8] Among women over sixty-five, 62 percent wanted to lose weight although 65 percent of them were not overweight. Women in my own practice tend to describe their own body features in comparison to what's being shown, which tends to be a younger ideal. Do you spend a lot of time comparing yourself to the models on magazine covers or to famous entertainers? How does it make you feel?

GET PAST YOUR PAST

Once you've developed a negative body image pattern, it becomes very powerful. It plays a role in how you feel about your body, how you see it, what you think about it, and how you behave in relation to it. You wind up perceiving yourself as unattractive regardless of reality. You may even reshape your experiences to fit your distorted view, noticing and remembering only negative comments and incidents involving your body.

But now that you know the factors that put you at risk for a negative body image, you can start working on a new image. Some of us have internalized negative messages about our body, identified with a parent who has a negative body image, and/or project onto our bodies negative feelings about ourselves, and all of us are affected by the culture. Regardless of which processes have impact on you, you can accept your body as a positive source of feelings, physical needs, and information about yourself. The next goal is to help you develop new, more positive ways to think about and treat your physical self. The chapters ahead will help you break out of your cage and create a healthier body image.

PART TWO

Reconstruct a Healthy Body Image in Midlife

3

SET A REALISTIC WEIGHT GOAL

[Wolves] all have their own body configurations and strengths, their own beauty. They live and play according to what and who and how they are. They do not try to be what they are not.

—Clarissa Pinkola Estes, Ph.D.,
Women Who Run with the Wolves

I see women coming in for treatment who used to be able to exercise three times a week, watch what they ate, and look the way that they wanted to look. Now as midlife and menopause kick in, all of a sudden what's worked before is no longer effective. These women, who tend to be very busy, respond by trying harder—and they're exhausted. It's very disheartening.

Do you identify with this scenario? Do you often find yourself telling your friends, "No matter what I do, I can't stay as slim as I used to?" Maybe it's time to think outside the cage and say, "Wait a minute. Is this drive to be as thin as I was when I was young a good idea? Maybe I'm aiming for something that isn't healthy, fulfilling, or life enhancing for a woman my age. Maybe my real power and appeal (sexual and otherwise) is going to come from owning who I am and where I am, and figuring out a way to be that will feel good. If I exercise and I can make love with my partner for hours, is that more important than looking like a teenage idol or fitting into the clothes that I wore at thirty?" Maybe it's time to donate those clothes and find new ones that really communicate something authentic about you as a woman of forty-five, fifty-five, or whatever your age.

WHAT'S ACHIEVABLE IN MIDLIFE?

You may say, "I want to wear a size six and weigh 108 pounds." But are you willing to work that hard and long—and eat so little? Do you want to get down to 108, only to wind up regaining the lost pounds again in a few months? Or could you accept wearing a size 10 and weighing 125 pounds? The drive to be thin leads many women to dieting that produces the yo-yo phenomenon, the body's ever increasing resistance to weight loss, and often an upwardly spiraling body weight. We know from research that when you continually diet and then regain weight, you add more fat.

Midlife women have grown up with a body shape ideal which is so thin that very few women can ever achieve it. Those who do achieve it tend to invest extraordinary amounts of time, energy, and resources—a difficult feat for most of us. The American ideal body shape for a female places us in a double bind because it's so extreme. It sets us up for failure. When we can't reach the weight target, we feel fat and beat ourselves up. Often we stigmatize ourselves with all the negative stereotypes associated with being fat. We put ourselves down as lazy and lacking willpower and self-control. It's a lose-lose situation that erodes most women's self-esteem—and it ignores the reality of a woman's body.

Body fat increases as you get older, and fat burns fewer calories than muscle. Metabolism slows down, making it more difficult to maintain weight or lose it. You've probably had a few kids, and your body shows it. Your belly sticks out. During perimenopause and menopause, changing estrogen levels cause fat to be redistributed in the waist and stomach area for many women. In order to reach today's standard of thinness despite such changes, you have to take measures that border on the unhealthy and cause incredible stress.

Heredity counts as well. Studies of weight control and setpoint theory (setpoint is a weight to which our body seems to return no matter how hard we try to lose more pounds) have demonstrated that our genetic inheritance plays a large part in our weight and distribution of fat in our bodies.[1] The book *Successful Aging* by John W. Rowe, M.D., and Robert L. Kahn, Ph.D., which presents results of the MacArthur Studies of Successful Aging, includes the finding that over two-thirds of the risk of obesity can be attributed to your genes. Women have been told that they can have a movie star figure if only they practice self-control, but the reality of genetic predisposition mandates that the current body ideal is unattainable for most of us.

Some people are going to gain weight easier than others, and some will find weight more difficult to take off than others. Let's say the women in your family of origin tend to have large frames and weigh 180 pounds. They eat normally, do not diet, and may not exercise. You will probably have a tougher time losing weight than someone from a family with a similar lifestyle, but where women weigh 150 pounds and have a medium frame.

Does that mean you're doomed to be fat? No, but it may mean you need to accept wearing clothes a size or two larger than your dream. If you base your self-worth on achieving the unachievable, you're likely to experience failure and challenges to your feelings of self-worth. That price is too high to pay—and unnecessary. Ironically, women often report that they want to lose weight to be more attractive to men. Yet research shows that when people are asked to pick out the most appealing females in a group, men choose those who are eleven to thirteen pounds heavier than women do. Men like slender women, but they also want breasts and curves.

YOUR REALISTIC GOAL WEIGHT

I'm going to challenge you to set a realistic goal weight rather than yo-yo back and forth for the rest of your life. That means a weight that is right for you—not a magazine model—and at which you can be successful. For example, I worked with a woman who had been a size 14 and slimmed down to a size 10. But she wanted to be a size 8. Ten was realistic, but 8 was not. To stay a 10, she had to exercise six times a week and curtail her food intake dramatically. If she consumed any fewer calories, she'd be famished—which would be a mistake. Research shows that when you overdo food restrictions, you tend to wind up bingeing in response to the starvation.

A realistic weight is one you can realistically achieve. Nothing is more motivating than success. A realistic weight is also one you can realistically maintain.

To determine your realistic weight, think in terms of weight ranges. Because factors such as age, body type, genetics, and medications play a role, there is no one number on a scale that fits all. Then look at your body mass index (BMI), which is the measurement of weight relative to height and is an estimate of body fat. BMI is the newest way of looking at weight. A normal BMI range is important because excess body fat increases your risk for diabetes, cardiovascular disease, hypertension, certain cancers, and other serious health problems. If extra fat is located around your waist—as opposed to thighs and buttocks—research suggests that your risk is even higher.

A BMI range between 18.5 kg/m and 24.9 kg/m is considered normal, but you shouldn't be in the low end of normal in your fifties and beyond. A BMI of 25 kg/m to 29.9 kg/m is considered overweight, and 30 kg/m and above is classified as obesity, according to the National Heart, Lung, and Blood Institute.

Check the chart to identify your BMI. If you are shorter than the heights shown or weigh more than the figures shown, you can

WEIGHT (lbs.)

HEIGHT	100	105	110	115	120	125	130	135	140	145	150	155	160	165	170	175	180	185	190	195	200	205	210	215	220	225	230	235	240	245	250
5'0"	20	21	21	22	23	24	25	26	27	28	29	30	31	32	33	34	35	36	37	38	39	40	41	42	43	44	45	46	47	48	49
5'1"	19	20	21	22	23	24	25	26	26	27	28	29	30	31	32	33	34	35	36	37	38	39	40	41	42	43	43	44	45	46	47
5'2"	18	19	20	21	22	23	24	25	26	27	27	28	29	30	31	32	33	34	35	36	37	37	38	39	40	41	42	43	44	45	46
5'3"	18	19	19	20	21	22	23	24	25	26	27	27	28	29	30	31	32	33	34	35	35	36	37	38	39	40	41	42	43	43	44
5'4"	17	18	19	20	21	21	22	23	24	25	26	27	27	28	29	30	31	32	33	33	34	35	36	37	38	39	39	40	41	42	43
5'5"	17	17	18	19	20	21	22	22	23	24	25	26	27	27	28	29	30	31	32	32	33	34	35	36	37	37	38	39	40	41	42
5'6"	16	17	18	19	19	20	21	22	23	23	24	25	26	27	27	28	29	30	31	31	32	33	34	35	36	36	37	38	39	40	40
5'7"	16	16	17	18	19	20	20	21	22	23	23	24	25	26	27	27	28	29	30	31	31	32	33	34	34	35	36	37	38	38	39
5'8"	15	16	17	17	18	19	20	21	21	22	23	24	24	25	26	27	27	28	29	30	30	31	32	33	33	34	35	36	36	37	38
5'9"	15	16	16	17	18	18	19	20	21	21	22	23	24	24	25	26	27	27	28	29	30	30	31	32	32	33	34	35	35	36	37
5'10"	14	15	16	16	17	18	19	19	20	21	22	22	23	24	24	25	26	27	27	28	29	29	30	31	32	32	33	34	34	35	36
5'11"	14	15	15	16	17	17	18	19	20	20	21	22	22	23	24	24	25	26	26	27	28	29	29	30	31	31	32	33	33	34	35
6'0"	14	14	15	16	16	17	18	18	19	20	20	21	22	22	23	24	24	25	26	26	27	28	28	29	30	31	31	32	33	33	34
6'1"	13	14	15	15	16	16	17	18	18	19	20	20	21	22	22	23	24	24	25	26	26	27	28	28	29	30	30	31	32	32	33
6'2"	13	13	14	15	15	16	17	17	18	19	19	20	21	21	22	22	23	24	24	25	26	26	27	28	28	29	30	30	31	31	32
6'3"	12	13	14	14	15	16	16	17	17	18	19	19	20	21	21	22	22	23	24	24	25	26	26	27	27	28	29	29	30	31	31
6'4"	12	13	13	14	15	15	16	16	17	18	18	19	19	20	21	21	22	23	23	24	24	25	26	26	27	27	28	29	29	30	30

Reprinted with permission from Shape Up America! www.shapeup.org

also calculate your BMI this way: (1) Multiply your weight in pounds by 703. (2) Then square your height in inches (for example, multiply 65 inches by 65 inches). (3) Divide the result of (1) by the result of (2). You can also use the BMI calculator at www.nhlbisupport.com/bmi/bmicalc.htm.

What is your BMI right now? Fill it in below:

My current BMI is: _____ kg/m

Is your BMI within the normal range—under 25? If so, you're at a healthy weight. If not, the ultimate goal is to reduce your BMI to below 25. How far away are you? How can you successfully get there?

Pamela Peeke, M.D., MPH, author of *Fight Fat After 40,* and a Pew Scholar in the Biomedical Sciences, advises you to aim to lose 10 percent of your body weight in pounds.

Fill in below:

My target loss is 10 percent of my weight: _____ pounds

For example, if you're five feet four and weigh 160, your BMI is 27. Plan to take off 10 percent of your weight, or sixteen pounds. That will take you down to 144 pounds, a BMI below 25. If you wish to go a bit lower to give yourself wiggle room, that's up to you.

What if 10 percent is too much? Then obviously you can lower it to 5 percent. The important thing is to develop more healthy lifestyle habits, eating right and exercising.

On the other hand, if the 10 percent loss is not enough to bring you to a normal BMI range, take one step at a time. If you're five feet four and weigh 180 pounds, your BMI is 31. Drop eighteen pounds (10 percent), and your BMI comes down to around 27. That's a good start. Then look at your ultimate goal (a BMI under 25) and fill in:

My ultimate weight loss target is: _____ pounds

Give yourself credit for what you've accomplished so far. A 10 percent loss is something to be proud of.

Realize that BMI guidelines are something to shoot for. Don't make them a standard that causes you to feel bad about yourself, because standards can change. The fact is, a few years ago, 27 was considered a normal BMI. And scientists are now investigating whether the cutoff for a normal BMI should vary according to ethnic group.

"People think they have to lose boatloads of weight, but the body is very forgiving. A 10 percent drop in weight can help reverse high blood pressure and diabetes—and it's a number that's achievable. Even if you weigh two hundred fifty pounds, 10 percent is only twenty five pounds," says Peeke.

"If you can't follow up the 10 percent with enough of a loss to reach the normal BMI range, that's fine as long as you got where you are the healthy way, eating sensibly and exercising. You have to be realistic and look at the genetic deck of cards you've been dealt. We all have different body frames and fat distribution. But you can make the most of what you have," says Peeke.

TIMING IS EVERYTHING

Once you've determined a realistic goal weight for yourself, the challenge is to develop a lifestyle to support it. If you find that you aren't losing the pounds or inches that you want, you need to change what you've done in the past. You can't get different results doing the same thing. For example, exercise is crucial to success. If you don't do any, you need to get moving. If you already exercise, you may need to add to it.

Don't attempt to reach your goal at a point when you've just taken on a huge work project or you're coping with a family crisis. It may be too difficult to find the time to exercise as you should or to concentrate on eating sensibly. Trying to lose weight when you don't have the time to do it right sets you up for failure.

Women tend to resist the reality of their time pressures, which only makes them feel stressed and frustrated. They'll say, "I have to be at my kids' sports and school events and I also have to take care of my elderly mother. She has cancer and has been given twelve months to live." At such times, maybe it's really important to be with your mother. If she's only going to live another year, maybe your goal must switch to: "I'm going to be a witness and honor her for this last year. Once that's over and I won't have to go to the nursing home three times a week, then I can take those three nights to work out."

Demands on our time tend to increase at midlife, and if that's what's going on for you, then losing weight may have to be postponed. You may choose to work on your weight at another time, or switch your goal to developing healthy eating habits, while eating moderately. This doesn't mean you are lazy. You truly don't have the time.

However, if you find that you never ever have time, then you need to stop and question why that is so. Why aren't you taking yourself seriously enough to make your own self-care a priority?

I once attended a talk by Stephan Rechtschaffen, M.D., author of *Timeshifting,* where he told a story about Gandhi. In my workshops I often share the story, which illustrates the importance of facing the truth and the role of timing.

Gandhi was leading a civil disobedience march to protest working conditions. One million people converged to join the march, and every day Gandhi meditated for guidance. One day he went to his lieutenants and announced, "I have meditated about this

*march, and we have to turn back. I know this is the wrong time."
Shocked, the lieutenants replied, "We're not turning back. These
people have left their lives to march. They've left their homes
and their work to fight for this cause. We can't just turn back."*

*Gandhi responded, "I've been meditating and I foresee that
there's going to be violence. This is not going to be effective. We
need to turn back." Again his lieutenants said, "We won't stop
now. These people have given up too much to follow you. What
will they think of you as a leader?"*

*Gandhi replied, "My commitment is to the truth, not con-
sistency."*

We all need to face and live with the truth, even when it's inconvenient or troublesome. But this is especially urgent for women,
who consistently overcommit themselves when attempting a
weight loss program. The result is that they fail. They then feel bad
about themselves, instead of facing the truth—that the reason
they haven't succeeded is that this might not be the right time to
try, and because there are too many other demands in their lives.

Instead of feeling inadequate, accept the fact that in order to
lose weight in midlife, you will have to make a considerable time
commitment. It involves cardiac workouts, strength training sessions, and the time to buy fresh food and prepare healthy meals.
It also requires time each day to relax, enjoy quiet time, and perhaps meditate, so that you do not respond to stress by overeating.
You may have to wait to do that. Otherwise you set yourself up
for failure and are likely to lament, "Other people can do it. Why
can't I?" The answer is, Because you don't have the resources. You
either have to make the time to do it right or not do it at all.

You are in charge of your life. You have a right to say, "I'm not
going to do that right now" or "I'm going to shoot for an inter-
mediate goal this year." However, continue to try to eat as healthy
as you can, of course, and continue to walk.

REJECT EXTREMES

Success in weight loss is the ability to achieve an appropriate weight in a way that you can maintain for life. In order to get out of the cycle of overeating and dieting, the key is to move your body—and we now have a plethora of wonderful new things to do, such as yoga, tai chi, and Pilates—and avoid extremism in exercise and eating. Forget fad diets and gimmicks. The majority of them make exaggerated promises, such as "lose twenty pounds in six days"; or they advise extreme measures, such as eat only cabbage soup. If something has not been tested in evidence-based medical literature, pass it up.

What nutrition plan should you follow? Go to the websites of respected health organizations such as the American Heart Association, which offers dietary guidelines and other information you can download, or the American Dietetic Association. Such organizations keep updating their information and have been around a long time, unlike others that come and go. If you're someone who needs face-to-face group support and accountability, a plan like Weight Watchers is healthy and works for many people.

Some women prefer to consult a nutritionist. That's fine as long as you check the person's credentials. You want either a registered dietitian (RD) or someone with a master's degree in nutrition (MS). Some dietitians have both credentials. For referrals, call the American Dietetic Association's National Center for Nutrition and Dietetics' Consumer Nutrition Hot Line (1-800-366-1655) or contact a local hospital and ask for someone who works with midlife women.

DON'T USE YOUR SCALE EVERY DAY

Reject extremes regarding the scale, as well. The scale is an important tool when used appropriately but not when you turn to it several times a day. To avoid torturing yourself, plan about four weigh-ins a month. Weigh yourself first thing in the morning, when you are naked, and after you've gone to the bathroom. If you do it at 4 P.M. or 7 P.M., you set yourself up for a letdown. "The average woman can gain three pounds of water weight a day just from eating," comments Peeke, who also advises taking your menstrual cycle into account if you still have one. Don't get on the scale when approaching or having your period, because you'll weigh more. The truest weight you can get is about ten days after the start of your menstrual cycle, if your cycle is fairly normal. If your menstrual cycle is irregular, or if you don't have one anymore, use the ring test. Take a favorite ring that usually fits fine. If you can't slip it on, you could be bloated—and therefore weigh more. Visit the scale when the ring fits.

LAURA'S SUCCESS STORY

Although Laura weighed 108 pounds when she got married after college, she crept up to 120 in her forties. After menopause, she continued to add weight, despite a low-fat diet and exercise three or four times a week. Always a size 6 or 8, she found herself to be a size 10. Then she inched up to a 12. "I joked that I'd have to start shopping for plus sizes. I needed a size 14 in pants because my stomach stuck out so much," she recalls. "I hated how I looked. I'd see pictures of my pudgy face and tell my husband, 'I look like a chipmunk.' I felt heavy and old-looking."

At five feet three inches tall, Laura couldn't believe that her weight crept up to 144 pounds (a BMI of 26). "I felt so helpless. I was already eating less fat and exercising more than any of my friends," she explains. Laura's sister-in-law, whom she hadn't seen in almost a year, came to dinner. "She had lost twenty pounds— and shared how much better she felt," says Laura. Laura told her about her dilemma with weight, and they discussed it.

Laura felt that she wanted to do it right, however, without pills of any kind or extreme regimens. She had come to realize that her low-fat eating plan didn't work because it ignored calories. She overdosed on bagels and pasta.

Laura's sister-in-law had successfully lost weight by following a diet provided by a hospital nutritionist. Laura decided to try it. Sensible and balanced, it helped her slim down over a four- to five-month period. "I wanted an eating regimen that I could live with forever, one where I could increase my calories somewhat after I reached my goal, but continue eating healthy and in moderation. It worked for me."

Laura figured out that 128 to 130 pounds was a reasonable weight that she could live with. It was low enough so that she would look good, but not so low that she'd have to starve or increase her exercise time, which was already substantial. She lost fifteen pounds, reaching her goal, and has maintained that weight for three years so far.

A big help has been a change in her attitude toward food. "I decided that food was too much of a focus of pleasure for me. Sure, I wanted to enjoy it, but I also had lots of other satisfactions and joys in life. I didn't want to give food such importance anymore."

If you want to take control and make food less powerful in your life, as Laura did, try this. Go to a party. Focus on the people you are with rather than the food on the buffet table. Loosen up and ask them questions about themselves, and share information about you. Be open to talking to other guests you haven't met before. What is that experience like for you? Do you find yourself having interesting conversations, meeting new people, and having fun? Do the people "fill you up"? Is there any difference in what and how much you eat?

EAT—DON'T STARVE

To succeed at your realistic weight goal, you not only need to take care of your body and feed it good food but you also have to be fair to it. The great majority of midlife women have been traumatized with diets for years, and the biggest mistake you can make is to find another short-term solution and revert to patterns that don't work. The most toxic behaviors when trying to lose weight are constant food restriction and meal skipping. When you starve your body, you only wind up bingeing because you're so hungry that you lose control. The best defense against overeating is to eat.

Here's another reason to eat, not starve. When a person begins to diet, the body interprets the lowered food intake as starvation. As a result, the metabolic rate slows down, and the body becomes more efficient, wasting less. Then when the individual begins to eat normally again, the body prepares for the next period of starvation by storing food as fat. And the cycle renews itself.

Women often tell me stories such as this one: "I've really been trying so hard to slim down. I only ate a piece of toast and juice for breakfast. I skipped lunch and thought, 'Good, I'll save calories.' When I got home, I hadn't eaten in eight hours. I started to make dinner, and I was munching on cheese and crackers. As I cut the salad, I ate pretzels. Then since I ate so much, I figured, 'What the heck' and let it rip. I ate some more." The woman will then insist, "I have no self-control." And I'll reply, "No, you have a lot of self-control. You run a business and you manage a household. But you were starving. You would have been much better off with a turkey sandwich at noon than the fifteen hundred calories you ate before sitting down to your evening meal."

Something similar recently happened in my own life. I expected to go out for dinner with my husband. Then I realized that the restaurant we love was closed that day, so I ran to the store to shop for ingredients for a quick supper. Once home, I put the chicken in the oven and got the rice cooking. But I wound up filling a big bowl with barbecued potato chips, which my kids and I devoured. It wasn't a smart move, but I was starving.

Laura took a much healthier approach when she found herself

starving at 5 P.M. one night, although her husband wasn't due home for dinner until 7 P.M. She usually feeds such hunger with an apple or a cup of plain nonfat yogurt, which allows her to wait for her meal. But this time, she wanted real food. She ate a portion of the turkey meat loaf she had prepared for dinner, despite worry that she'd then eat a second portion later when she sat down with her husband. It didn't work out that way. "After eating early, I felt satisfied," she explains. "I didn't want more meat loaf at 7 P.M. I had enough. I felt perfectly fine eating just the side vegetables I'd prepared. That was all I needed."

Laura's experience is a great example of listening to your internal signals. If you pay attention to your hunger when you feel it, and respond to it, you don't have to worry about bingeing. The binge simply won't happen because the body doesn't need the calories.

Laura also avoids overeating at parties by eating a small amount before she goes. If a dinner party is scheduled for 7:30 P.M. and she knows that food won't be served until 8:00 or 8:30, she eats something at home first, when she's hungry. A piece of turkey on a small salad or some cheese on a rice cake are good choices at such times. Then she winds up wanting only a small amount at the party. "If I show up starving, I'm a goner, especially after having a glass of wine," she says.

For long-term weight loss and maintenance, eating when the body asks to be fed and making your food choices as healthy as possible are key. Remember, eating prevents overeating—don't starve yourself.

ACCEPT YOUR LOSS

It's hard to accept that you're never going to have the body you had, or weigh what you did, in your twenties. Yet when you surrender to reality, it opens a whole new world of options, energy, and joy. You grow by confronting your limits. When I talk about realistic weight in my workshops, I often discuss some of the principles of Buddhism to illustrate how liberating it can be to let go of an unattainable body ideal. Buddhism is the religion founded by the great religious teacher Buddha. Buddha's doctrine holds that pain is part of life. It's not due to the fact that you didn't meditate enough or did something wrong. It is simply part of the human condition.

The principle map that Buddha used to teach about the journey to happiness is called the Four Noble Truths. For our purposes, we'll explore the first two noble truths. The First Noble Truth is that pain is inevitable. Life is painful because life is, by nature, difficult. Pain is inherent because everything in life is always changing. Illness and death are painful.

The Second Noble Truth is that suffering is optional. We can't help that there is pain in our lives, but we can choose whether to suffer or not suffer. Suffering occurs when we struggle against our life experience (i.e., that everything changes) instead of accepting and opening ourselves to it.

The positive aspect of everything always changing is that if you're in a bad place, the bad times won't last forever. They will change. It's very comforting for people to hear that. Conversely, if you're in a good place in your life, you should really enjoy it, because you won't always be in that place. Changes go on all around you. Your body gets older, your kids leave, companies lay off people. If you refuse to accept that reality and deal with it, you suffer.

Another source of suffering that Buddha talked about is craving what you can't have, for example, pleasure, money, or youth. When you crave a body that is just not possible anymore, you're choosing suffering.

What would happen if you let go of that craving, and instead said, "I'm going to try to eat really healthy. I'm going to try to exercise, get some great clothes, and accept that I'm going to be a size 12. There is enough suffering in midlife. I don't need to choose this type of suffering anymore."

SANDY'S SUCCESS STORY

Sandy, an attractive, vibrant woman of fifty-five, has accepted that you can't stop the clock. She recalls, "It was really hard in my forties to look at my body and to see that it was getting older and wider." Oddly enough, her thinking changed after a drastic alteration in her lifestyle sent her into deep depression. Sandy and her family had lived a life of luxury in Brazil until an economic downturn put her husband's construction business into bankruptcy. The family migrated to the United States to start all over again. However, anticipated business connections never materialized. Accustomed to being waited on by maids, Sandy found herself living in a middle-class neighborhood in New Jersey, struggling to make ends meet. The social support she had enjoyed from relatives and friends was left behind. During this period, her father and sister also died. Crushed by loss, she couldn't get out of bed in the morning.

"My sister-in-law saved my life," she says. "She came over every day to help with the children and talk to me about how much I had to live for and be grateful for. She pulled me out of it." Sandy emerged from her depression finally accepting her new circumstances and ready to get on with her life. She also stopped fighting her body.

"Now in my fifties, I've come to accept that aging is inevitable. I choose to love my body, love myself, and to enjoy all the good things in my life. My children live nearby. I have two wonderful grandchildren. Yes, I have lines in my face and I've gained thirty-five pounds. I will not be skinny again. But I look pretty good. I wear nice clothes and I pick out flattering colors.

"My knee is starting to bother me and my son told me, 'Ma, you have to do exercise because you can't let that go.' I never exercised before, but I now do it five times a week. I feel much better. I have to take care of my health."

Sandy got over the rough adjustment from South America to

the United States, making the transition into midlife with self-care and determination. When she stopped craving what she couldn't have—her old life of privilege and her younger body—she felt enormously free. She accepted that everything changes and that change doesn't have to be negative.

TAKING UP SPACE

Some women have a very hard time reaching acceptance. When I work with midlife women who are binge eaters, I find that they often have lost and regained weight over the years and so are storing more fat. Often they want to lose more weight than is possible. I particularly remember one group of women who were really stuck. They kept insisting on returning to what they weighed when they were in their twenties, before they had children. I told them I was concerned that they were setting an unrealistic goal, and that in order to reach it they'd have to eat so little that they'd eventually begin to overeat again. That wasn't a smart way to go. To help them develop a more realistic goal weight and realize what they were doing to themselves, I asked them to try an exercise.

I said, "I want each of you to find a space in this room that is too small for your body or a part of your body, such as under a chair or in between bookcases, or between the lamp and the wall. I want you to squeeze into that space, even though it might actually hurt to fit into it."

I then added, "I want you to pay attention to how your body feels, and how you feel. Speak up and tell us." Soon after, a few began to report, "My leg is hurting; the arm of the chair is sticking in my knee." Or, "I'm getting a bruise on my arm." I repeated these statements to the group. This set off a spirited discussion, because the women really had squeezed themselves into the spaces. They had marks on their bodies, and they felt physically uncomfortable. Their initial comments expanded to, "We do this all the time. We always try to make ourselves into what other people want, whether we fit or not." One woman finally said, "I can't stand this. This is what my life is like. I'm always trying to fit into other people's expectations, to become a body shape I can't fit. It hurts a lot, just like right now I have a big red bruise on my leg. I'm getting out of this space."

Women are often taught, "You're a good woman if you're able to tolerate being uncomfortable and sculpting your body and self into what others want you to be. You're noble, strong, and disciplined if you can whip your body into a size 6." But it's not possible for most women to do that. It takes courage to go inside and figure out what truly is realistic for you, instead of what your mother or children or lover say you should look like.

DEVELOP A NEW KIND OF POWER

According to our media and our culture, the definition of power is beauty and the ability to make your body ultrathin. Women have been encouraged to look outside themselves for what is considered beautiful and thus powerful. But we must challenge ourselves to grow a new kind of power—intrinsic power, which is a feeling of potency and competence in the world. That kind of power can be strengthened by defining yourself clearly, and knowing what you value in life, as well as in your appearance.

J. Rotter, a research psychologist, argued that people's attitudes could be placed along a continuum ranging from seeing what happens to them as being under their control to seeing what happens to them as being under the control of external forces. At one end of this continuum there are those who are internally oriented, believing that events and consequences are largely under their control. At the opposite end are people who are externally oriented. They generally believe that there's little they can do to influence events in their life and that events are the result of luck, chance, or fate. Rotter called this personality characteristic *locus of control.*

One study[2] found that women who had an internal locus of control tended to have more positive attitudes toward their body images. They were more likely to endorse feelings of physical attractiveness, strength, and fitness, and less likely to endorse feelings of disparagement about their bodies. On the other hand, women who had a more external locus of control were more likely to feel fat and negative toward their bodies and to consider body shape and weight more important in their lives. These women were less likely to endorse feelings of attractiveness, physical strength, and fitness.

Do you feel that you have control over your life—or does it seem as if outside forces define you? To achieve healthy power, you need to develop a more internal locus of control. The thermostat or compass of direction has to be inside of you, not outside of you. Women who set their own agenda, whatever their age, have the most success.

Take Chris, sixty, a controller for a Los Angeles toiletries wholesaler. Born in Trinidad, Chris is five feet two inches tall, has a medium frame, and weighs 150 pounds. When she looks in the mirror, she says, "I feel good. I don't feel my age. At times I see a vein I didn't have before or a new wrinkle, but I'm comfortable in my body even though I gained thirty pounds in my fifties. My bra size is much bigger now and I don't wear certain things because I'm too busty. I do think, 'Why did all the weight have to go there?' I know I have to minimize it and change the way I dress. I don't wear low-cut blouses or strapless tops like I used to. They make me look too big on top. I see the changes in my body, but I think I'm attractive. I am eating healthy and have an active lifestyle. I feel good."

You can reject what is supposedly a correct body type as Chris did, finding direction within yourself and accepting your body changes through the seasons of your life. You can stop compulsive weigh-ins, and using tape measures as compasses. What is normal at one age may be unrealistic at another.

Power is not sculpting yourself into a cover girl. Power is looking within and developing your own ideal body—which is based on genetics, bone structure, age, and the amount of time you can devote to exercise.

The alternative is unhappiness. Often a midlife woman will come into my office and say, "I think I'm depressed. Nothing seems that exciting to me." As I talk to her, it becomes apparent how much her focus and worry about her body failing to reach the ideal of thinness diminishes her zest for life and her general contentment, even though she may feel good about herself in other ways that have nothing to do with appearance. My colleague psychologist Ruth Striegel-Moore, Ph.D., labels this worry about appearance, which most women feel to some degree, *normative discontent.*

Normative discontent can even take on a moral tone. Weight prejudice has become a social norm. The person who is fat in this country is viewed as morally lazy. One patient I worked with told me, "Being overweight is bad, and in some ways that makes me a bad person and a less worthwhile person." This view gets associated with thoughts such as, "I don't have self-control," or "I'm out of control." It virtually becomes an indictment of the person's integrity or strength of character. Normative discontent strikes very admirable women who raised great kids, are moving ahead in their careers, and/or are active members of the community. The attitude is extremely troubling. Let's change it and begin to reclaim your power by setting a weight target that you can really achieve and really maintain. Remember, this is not the weight you were at twenty, but rather the weight that works for you at midlife.

4

BEAT EMOTIONAL EATING

For me, it works better to give food and hunger a space in my life, but in a friendly way so that I don't destructively devour twelve cookies at a time.

—Natalie Goldberg,
Writing Down the Bones

You spend the afternoon chauffeuring the kids to soccer practice and gymnastics, and visiting and shopping for your father, who is seriously ill but insists on remaining in his apartment without help. When you get home, you grab an almost-full can of cashew nuts and consume it all. Or when traveling on business, your connecting flight gets canceled; stuck in the airport for four hours waiting for the next available plane, you head for the fast-food counters to pig out on pizza and donuts. Or when you are unable to sleep, you get up in the middle of the night and attack a pint of chunky chocolate nut premium ice cream.

Do you often find yourself in such situations? Do you know all about good nutrition—what you should and shouldn't put into your body—yet find yourself eating cookies instead of grapes when you want a snack? Do you understand why? The fact is, many of us eat for emotional reasons rather than to satisfy feelings of genuine hunger. According to the Calorie Control Council, 28 percent of dieters say they fail because of frequent emotional eating.

People generally succumb to emotional eating for three reasons:

1. To handle difficult emotional states, such as fatigue, deprivation, or frustration.
2. To fill needs unmet by other people in their lives.
3. They aren't eating enough.

In my practice, I often help clients explore these issues and look at practical ways to deal with them. You can learn to deal with them, too.

HANDLING DIFFICULT EMOTIONAL STATES

We know from research that when you're fatigued or deprived, whether of food, recognition, or help when you need it, your ability to regulate your emotions and make healthy choices declines. Our exhausted society, with our twelve-hour workdays and multiple responsibilities for caring for elders, children, and household, is a setup for unhealthy choices, especially when it comes to food. You may be too tired when you come home to say no to cheesecake.

Feelings of deprivation may also lead you to overeat or select high-fat, high-calorie foods. If you feel deprived, it can mean that you haven't eaten enough food today and you're starving or that you haven't had enough downtime to refuel and refresh yourself. Your ability to make good food decisions decreases after a long, intense day.

Let's say you're a teacher. You spent the day in the classroom. Then you followed it up by going to your own kids' music recital. Since none of you had time for dinner, you all stopped on the way home to eat at a local diner. You walk in the house at 10 P.M., and the first thing you notice is the laundry basket overflowing. You can hardly stand on your feet, and your mind feels like mush. If you were thinking clearly and weren't so fatigued, you might say to yourself, "The laundry will be here tomorrow. I'll get my husband and the kids to help me with it then. Right now I'm going straight to bed." Instead, because you're tired, you'll probably fall into another mode, insisting, "I have to get this done tonight."

You load the laundry and wait for the washer to finish so that you can transfer the contents into the dryer. As you wait, you probably feel frustrated. Then you might find yourself opening the cabinet door to reach for the chocolate chip cookies or a bag of pretzels—even though you know that's not what you need. You might do so despite an awareness that you're not hungry.

Sound familiar? Women say to me all the time, "I knew I shouldn't have eaten those cookies even before I put them in my mouth, but I had to do it anyway. There's something wrong with me." I always urge them to leave judgment at the door and answer, "It does not mean that something is wrong with me. It does mean that my demands on myself are too high and my resources to cope are too low. Let me take a look at what happened today and what might have led to the binge." As they reconstruct their activities, they almost always find a tough situation they faced that day—and find some compassion for themselves. All of us will sometimes surrender to temptation when life is so hectic. Some stressed people tend to be night foragers because they finally have five seconds to themselves and want to inappropriately reward themselves for the exhaustion of the day. To numb themselves or help themselves feel better, some people eat a bunch of snacks. You're not "bad" for doing so, you're human, and your lifestyle may simply be too demanding. It's time to learn to change it.

DON'T FIGHT IT

As adults, when demands on us are too high and resources are too low, we leave the situation mentally or emotionally. We space out in front of the TV set or we eat or we drink until we're not really there. In contrast, a child tends to physically exit the situation, as my youngest son, Jonathan, did when faced with this stressful scenario at age four. At that time, my two oldest children played recreational soccer, and both of their teams were in the league championships that fall. The whole family was going to watch, including my father, who was flying in from Philadelphia. It was early in the morning, still dark in October, as my husband and I tried to get everyone ready to pick up my dad at the airport and head for the game. Jonathan is a child who needs time to wake up in the morning and must have something to eat before he gets moving. But we were in a hurry.

I woke him up, and he was cranky. He took his time getting dressed, then he wanted to eat. I told him, "You can have cupcakes, donuts, hot chocolate, anything you want when we get to the field, except for cereal." He insisted on cereal. My husband quickly said, "Okay, take a bag of cereal along in the car." But Jonathan wanted milk. "There's no time to sit down and eat it with milk. You have to get with the program," I said.

Quietly he announced, "I'm leaving." And nobody paid attention.

Later, out in the garage as we got into the car, my husband turned to me and asked, "Do you have Jonathan?"

I answered, "No, I thought you did."

When my husband ran into the house, Jonathan wasn't there. Then all of a sudden he appeared, walking down the driveway crying. He was leaving. He'd been forced to get up before dawn, jump out of bed, and give up the breakfast he wanted. And the resources he'd ordinarily have—organized, empathetic, thoughtful parents—weren't there. So he was getting out.

For Jonathan, the demands were too high, and the resources were missing. Children have different temperaments. It was wishful thinking for me to suppose that he'd just rush along with the rest of us. When I realized that the schedule was too much for him, I switched gears. I told my husband, "You take the kids to the game. I'll give Jonathan his breakfast. If I'm late to pick up my father, he's a grown-up and will understand. We'll get to the game when we get there."

Just as I should have paid attention to Jonathan's nature, it's also important for women to pay attention to their own natures. When we don't, we pay a high price. I recall one day, for example, when a flight I was taking left late for a business trip to Washington. I got to the hotel late, after having had only a soda and peanuts on the plane. I'm someone who has to eat each meal. If I don't, I can't function at my best.

By the time I got to my meeting, I felt very agitated and had developed a headache from not eating. At the end of the meeting I felt foggy. I stopped at a vending machine to buy cheese and crackers, which helped. But I asked myself, "Why didn't I stop off first to get something to eat, and go to the meeting a little late?" I would have felt better mentally and physically and performed better. Delayed flights happen, and people would have understood that there was snow in Cincinnati. Next time I'll get to the meeting an hour later, but I'll be more productive because I'll get something to eat first.

How often do you ignore your nature and respond to the demands of others the way I did? Are you open to change?

FIND A BALANCE

We are all trying to find a balance between the demands in our lives and our resources to deal with them. Anytime you know the healthy thing to do but can't do it, it's a red flag sign that you need to either decrease the demands on yourself or increase your resources.

To do that, take an inventory. Write down the demands in your life in the column at left. They might include: earning enough to help pay the kids' tuition, carpooling, taking responsibility for your elderly aunt who lives in a nursing home, supervising your recently widowed mother-in-law's medical needs, entertaining a client (or your husband's client), working overtime, or coordinating the renovation of the kitchen.

DEMANDS VS. RESOURCES	
Demands	Resources

Now, in the column at right, list the resources you have to deal with demands. Resources are sources of concrete help, such as a neighbor always available to babysit or an inheritance someone just left you, as well as enjoyable activities that help reduce the tension you're under. Time with friends, exercise, meditation, and involvement in a spiritual community, such as your church, are all resources. Now take a look. Is the demand column longer than the resource column? Are you working too many hours? Do you have too many responsibilities?

When stresses outnumber resources, symptoms like overeating or drinking appear. The purpose of these symptoms is to modulate the pain of an unbalanced lifestyle. To avoid the symptoms and prevent them from escalating, you need to make changes. You need to decide on ways to either decrease the demands on you or increase your resources. Otherwise you will continue to engage in unhealthy behaviors in an attempt to numb the pain of living this way.

A few years ago, I worked with a client who was able to make changes to cope with a heartbreaking home situation. Sophie was a forty-seven-year-old internist who found herself living a nightmare when her husband, also a physician, developed early Alzheimer's at age fifty-three. She started drinking wine every night and overeating for the first time in her life. She binged from the moment she got home until she went to bed, gaining twenty-four pounds in nine months.

When she first came to my office, she had tried several diet books to no avail. She couldn't stop eating. I asked her to compare the demands on her life at this tragic time with her resources. It became clear that the demands were crushing her. She had to maximize her income to meet the house payments, since her husband could no longer work. Plus, college tuition loomed ahead for their two teenage children. As a result, she had to put in longer hours in her practice at the same time that demands at home were agonizing and exhausting. Her husband, who used to be a resource, had moved over into the demand column.

In response to overwhelming demands in their lives, some people medicate themselves by overeating. Or they start yelling at everyone or begin to have two martinis each night. Alcohol reduces your inhibitions, which opens the door to bingeing. Because Sophie's life had become so stressful, she'd turned to food and wine.

I advised Sophie to reduce the demands on herself or increase her resources to relieve her symptoms. Her first reaction was, "I can't take a single thing off the demand list." But I suggested that we brainstorm some options. After talking for a while, she proposed, "Well, what if I make lower house payments?" Often reducing demands on yourself means giving something up—a big house, in her case. What you gain in mental and physical health far exceeds the trade-off.

All of our hard work together paid off for Sophie, leading her to make changes that increased her resources. She decided to put her house on the market and move to a smaller, less expensive one. The move reduced her monthly mortgage payments. And after she paid the down payment for her new home, she still had a lump sum of cash left over from the proceeds of her old house.

She became more involved in her synagogue, which offered a spiritual community she could tap for support and perspective. She treated herself to massages twice a month, which allowed her to be the one taken care of for a while. One night a week she went out to dinner or a movie with friends, who not only brought some laughter into her life but also provided empathy for her situation and a kind of emotional refuge.

Do you have to increase your resources or decrease demands on you before you can stop overeating or engaging in some other harmful behavior? What changes can you make? Are you giving too much and getting back too little?

Women in our society are taught the deprivation model—you're a good woman if you get by with less than you need. Many midlife women grew up with the TV show *Queen for a Day,* which glorified women as martyrs. Being a drudge and ignoring your own needs was considered a badge of honor. The trouble is, this kind of thinking leads women to feel exhausted—and often to turn to substances such as food for relief. We need to feel comfortable taking care of ourselves, which enables us to love and take good care of others in our lives. Putting your own needs first at times isn't selfish; it's necessary to give you the physical and emotional stamina to be there for those you care about.

FILLING UNMET NEEDS

Proponents of a psychoanalytic theory called *object relations* believe that the self, your ongoing sense of the essential qualities of who you are and how you fit into the world, develops through relationships with other people. We aren't born with a self, they say; we build one through sustained, meaningful connections, beginning with our primary caretaker and extending to other significant figures in our life.

Object relations theory views any mental disturbance, such as an eating disorder, as an attachment disturbance. When some individuals don't get their needs for love, dependence, or acceptance met by the people in their lives, they turn to an inanimate object outside the self—such as food or alcohol or drugs—to fulfill their needs. In other words, if you're overeating, sometimes it's because you're unable to engage others in gratifying relationships. You turn to food because you learned early in life that people are undependable, toxic, or dangerous.

Object relations theory helps me understand the problems that my clients struggle with. Someone will explain, "I can turn to food twenty-four hours a day. It never says no. I can depend on it to taste good. It's not going to bite back and say, 'You're too needy.' "

If you're having trouble with food, you may be someone who turns to eating because relationships haven't worked for you in the past—or because people have felt dangerous to you. I believe you can't develop a good relationship with food until you also develop a good relationship with your own body and with other people. People often feed or starve themselves in the manner in which they operate in daily life. For example, if you can never say no to people, you also may be unable to refuse food when you are no longer hungry.

I remember a patient who turned to food as a way to get nurturance without risking vulnerability, which is a necessary element in human relationships. For Caroline, fifty-five, who grew up in an affluent family, loving food was safer than loving people. Everyone important to her, beginning with her parents, failed her. Her father, with whom she had a poor relationship, was a workaholic; her mother was a perfectionist. Her first marriage ended in divorce, and her second marriage was unhappy as well. Others didn't meet her needs.

Caroline, who had a long history of using food to cope with transitions and separations, started overeating and drinking again when her daughter left for college. She wouldn't turn to her husband or friends for support because she struggled with being vulnerable in any way. Terrified that people wouldn't be there for her, she couldn't handle the possibility of disappointment.

Drinking became so important that she couldn't wait until 9 P.M. to start. Because she couldn't wait for meals either, she ate in between. At these times, she felt totally secure and safe. She didn't have to risk rejection from others. I told her, "It's as if your need for nurturance is met, but you're totally in control. You buy the food and wine, prepare it, and consume it."

In our work together, we discussed her lifelong focus on food, which relieved her from facing the disappointment that came from knowing she couldn't fix her parents and that she couldn't fix the emotionally unavailable men she picked as partners. Food kept Caroline filled up and safe. In order to change her eating and drinking habits and her life, Caroline had to take risks and allow herself to be vulnerable.

KNOW YOUR JOB DESCRIPTION

In order to develop a healthy relationship with food, you must develop a healthy relationship with your own body and with other people. All of these relationships have to change at the same time to make the changes last. If you just go on a diet for a month, you might lose some weight. But if you haven't dealt with the fact that you constantly overschedule yourself and that you're always exhausted because you do too much for other people and you're not getting your needs met, you're going to eventually start overeating again. The weight loss won't last. That's where a job description comes in. It requires you to sit down and think about where you need to say no. Remember that when you feel deprived or fatigued, your ability to make healthy decisions decreases.

Most women have great trouble saying no. They'll tell me, "I don't know when to say no to my kids." Or, "Am I being selfish if I don't pick up a friend at the airport, even though I'll have to turn myself into a wreck to do it?" Or, "I don't want to spend all day Saturday with my mother, but how can I refuse?" That's when thinking about your job description is really important.

I'll ask workshop participants, "What do you think is done in companies when you take a job? There's a job description, which outlines the boundaries of what you're supposed to do. As a daughter, what do you think your job description is?" Or, "What do you think your job description is as the mother of a twenty-two-year-old son? What are you supposed to do and what do you not need to do?" Or, "What is your job description as the wife of a fifty-six-year-old man?"

Women will talk about it, and someone might say, "I realize that I'm doing too much for my twenty-two-year-old son. If I stopped cleaning his room and doing his laundry and tell him it's his responsibility, that would free up three hours a week when I could exercise."

One mother, a fifty-two-year-old divorced nurse who has two college-age children living at home, said, "I still feel I have to come home from work to make dinner. I thought to myself the other day, 'It's so beautiful out. I would love to sit outside on the deck and read a book. I could just have cheese and crackers, some wine, some fruit.' But I feel trapped, like I have to come home and cook. Everyone expects it."

That's when I asked, "What's your job description with two college kids at home?" As we talked, it became clear that it didn't include making dinner every single night. The insight was very freeing for her. She decided then to go home and tell her children, "Monday, Wednesday, and Thursday I'm going to make dinner. Other nights, one of you make dinner or get take-out food, because I'm getting older and I really like sitting out there on the deck. I love that time of night when it cools off a little." Such a declaration is liberating, because women often allow the world to write their job descriptions for them.

Remember, too, that job descriptions can change as your life changes. Maybe you were someone who started out in a very traditional marriage and cooked dinner each night, but more money is available now. You can afford to go out to dinner two nights a week. Maybe your husband is willing and able to help out more. If you don't ask him, you'll never know.

IDENTIFY RELATIONSHIPS THAT MAKE YOU HUNGRY

To help women in my workshops focus not on dieting but on getting to the bottom of key relationship issues that keep them overeating, I ask the questions below. Try answering them for yourself.

1. Who are the three most important people in your life? Describe the frequency of contact.

2. Describe your expectations of close relationships with others. If the expectations are not fulfilled, what do you do? How do you eat before you see the people you're close to, while you're with them, and afterward?

3. Describe satisfying and unsatisfying aspects of your key relationships. How are you deliberate about making your relationships more satisfying?

4. What roles do you tend to play in relationships with others? Do certain roles leave you hungrier than others?

LOOKING AT YOUR ANSWERS

1. Your answer to this question will help you look at how close you really are to people. Sometimes a client will name the three most important people in her life—and it turns out that two of them live on the opposite coast. She sees them twice a year. She begins to realize that she really doesn't feel that close to them in daily life—and that lack of connection may be contributing to her obsession with eating.

    As we talk, she sees that she needs to develop closer relationships with people nearer to home. I suggest that she identify one coworker and one neighbor she'd like to know better and propose they go out to lunch or see a movie together.

2. How do you behave when you are disappointed? My client Diane felt devastated when her husband left her with three children. Divorced for three years, she finally started exercising and felt ready to date. But there was no guy. She told me, "I'm afraid that when I finally do meet someone I'll be so ready and so needy that I'll turn him off." I often hear about this fear from people who overeat. Many have had lives that have left them emotionally deprived.

    To help them control neediness, I ask them to picture an IV and think of it as a metaphor. Then I say, "You might think you need the whole IV bottle, and even deserve it. But the reality is that you're only going to get intermittent drips from the IV, rather than a constant flow. The focus has to move from 'How do I get all this attention from this person?' to 'How do I become skilled at getting drips so that I don't feel so deprived? I can't help that when I was younger I was deprived, but I am in charge now.'"

    When I used this technique on the divorcée, she came up with her own idea. "There is a singles volleyball team that I can join," she said. "Maybe just being around men, and exercising and sweating together, could be a drip. I could be with men in a fun way."

    She also came up with another great option. She missed having someone around to touch her, since she didn't have a lover. She and her sixteen-year-old daughter decided to give each other a manicure and pedicure once a month. The touch was great for them, and it was fun having downtime together. She found that the more she could get drips of self-care, the less she was prone to overeating.

3. The reality is people can never be there for you 24/7, but they can be there some of the time and you can get your needs met in measured doses. You may not be able to be the center of your mother's attention at the family picnic, telling her stories about your kids and your husband's new job, but you can invite her to lunch where the two of you

can focus on each other. Give your mom time to tell you what's important to her, too. There's a great feeling that comes from mutual interest and support in relationships. There are lots of different ways to get attention so that you don't wear one person out. For example, you may have had a difficult time at the office and you want to call your best friend to talk about it. Since you tend to complain about work a lot, it's helpful to set a time limit. You can say, "I'd like to take ten minutes to discuss what happened to me at the office today. Then I'll stop, and you take ten minutes to tell me what is on your mind."

To fulfill your need for human connection you must give up the illusion "I can always be gratified." You must also clearly ask for what you want.

4. At midlife, some women stand back and say, "Do I have to be the one who makes everybody smile? It's exhausting and draining." Are you the one who always has to listen and encourage—and does it leave you feeling tired because you have to be everyone's cheerleader? If you play a role where you constantly give and don't get much back, you can find yourself in the kitchen eating because you're feeling hungry to be taken care of.

I have a patient, a forty-three-year-old college professor, who realized that the reason she ate so much at night was that she was hungry from all the caretaking she did throughout the day. She lived with a man who'd fathered her two preschoolers. Although she knew he might leave her someday, she hadn't wanted to find herself old and childless. She went to parenting workshops, read books about child care, took her kids on interesting excursions on weekends, and was a very positive and encouraging mother. But her boyfriend wanted the same kind of nurturing energy from her, which was exhausting. She had the energy to be a cheerleader for her daughters, but she had none left at 9 P.M. for him. When you do too much nurturing, you tend to develop a hunger for care for yourself, which can be confused with hunger for food. Her response was to head for the kitchen for crackers, dip, and cheese.

I encouraged her to talk to her boyfriend and be specific about what she needed from him at 9 P.M., which was to snuggle and listen to the news or music together. It was also important to ask what she could do for him after the kids went to bed. He wanted her to rub his back and listen as he talked about his day. They negotiated that each would get a half hour of what they wanted every night.

STOP TRYING TO CHANGE PEOPLE

Many women spend a lot of time signaling people that they must change—that if they do so, everyone will be happier all around. But those you are trying to change may be people who are never going to change. You can continue to be stuck trying to change them, and out of frustration reach for the pistachio ice cream, or you can move in a new direction.

Susan, a divorced forty-six-year-old, successfully stopped trying to change her boyfriend. I remember her tearfully sharing the following story during her fourth therapy appointment with me.

Tom, the man she had been seeing exclusively for eight years, attended her professional organization's dinner dance. When the sixties' rock-and-roll music began to play, she purred, "I just love this song. Would you dance this one with me?"

He declined with, "You know I don't like to dance."

She told him it would mean a lot to her if they could dance together, but he shrugged and looked away. Then he turned to talk to a woman sitting next to him.

Feeling angry and frustrated, Susan ordered another glass of wine. Then she got up and went to the ladies' room. On her way back to the table, she saw him dancing with the other woman. She finished her apple tart for dessert and ate Tom's too. They left early and went to her home. After Tom fell asleep, she found her-self finishing up the pretzels in the cupboard.

"If only he would make a commitment to our relationship, be more nurturing and less self-centered, my life would be better," she told me. Tom had never had children and had never learned to put someone else's needs before his own, she added. "I've gained twenty-two pounds since I started dating him. He's affect-ing my eating and drinking, and it's all his fault. He still says he's not ready to ask me to marry him or become more involved with my kids as I would like. He won't go to their games or allow them to come along on vacation with us. When is he going to 'get it'? I can't move on with my life until he changes."

I shared with Susan my opinion that she had to make a decision. For eight years she had blamed him for her unhappiness. She was overeating, drinking too much at times, and losing confidence in herself. She had to either accept that this was all that Tom was will-ing to give—and enjoy it—or end the relationship. He had made it clear that he was not ready to get married and that he enjoyed see-ing her kids periodically but did not want to take on more of a par-enting role. "He's forty-one, never married, and is used to doing what he wants when he wants," Susan said sadly. She realized that she felt deprived in the relationship and had begun to turn to food and drinking instead of expecting him to meet her needs.

After that session, Susan began to realize that if Tom was not interested in negotiating a committed relationship with her, she would have to move on without him. "It may be painful without him," she said, "but I am realizing how painful it is with him. I have to take responsibility for my own happiness."

Later, Susan told me, "I was set on getting him to change. It was a rude awakening when I realized in that session that the only person I can change is myself."

Susan did change, giving Tom an ultimatum. When he hedged, she ended the relationship. Then she took other action. She got a personal trainer and began to work out regularly. She told me, "As my muscles get stronger, I feel stronger. I even leave my business forty-five minutes earlier so I can shop for fresh vegetables for myself." She started losing weight, and her body took on definition. She felt clearer about decisions at work and about her expectations of her two teenage daughters, whom she had always tended to be too easy on. She also changed socially. "I'm going out with a lot of friends, and instead of drinking, I just have club soda," she noted.

Later I learned that Susan went with some girlfriends on a trip to Hawaii, where she met a wonderful man—a doctor, who was also on vacation. They married within the year, and she moved to the East Coast.

Many women spend a lot of time telling others that they must change, but they may not be people who are going to change. You can continue to be stuck and reach for donuts—or try a new direction. Do you relate to Susan's experience? Are you trapped in the belief that once your husband or children or parents or friends change, your life will be happier? Do you put a lot of your energy and time into trying to change significant others in your life? Does it work? Do you wind up overeating, drinking, or shopping to avoid peering into the foggy places in your life and dealing with your own issues? What changes do you have to make to avoid turning to food instead of people for fulfillment?

LEARN TO TOLERATE EMPTINESS

Many people who overeat say, "I don't know why I do it. I'm just bored." Our culture of instant gratification views boredom and emptiness as conditions to be eliminated or fixed. When we experience these feelings, we rush away from them so very quickly by picking up a martini or diving into the lasagna.

In his book *Going to Pieces Without Falling Apart,* Mark Epstein, M.D., contrasts the Western view of emptiness as a torturous state to be avoided with the Buddhist perspective. Buddhists view feelings of emptiness as part of the fabric of everyday life. Emptiness doesn't have to be fixed because it's a natural state. It's part of life and the psyche—and if you can just stay with it, it will be transformed. It will often lead us to new meaning.

It is only when we stop fearing and fighting our personal emptiness that we can begin to appreciate that transformation is possible. If we don't allow ourselves to feel it, we don't learn and build character. We engage in all kinds of behaviors, such as eating, drinking, or spending too much money, to numb ourselves—and then we feel depressed because we still feel empty. Acting to avoid emptiness keeps us stuck. As a Buddhist teacher says in Epstein's book, "Learn to tolerate nothingness and your mind will be at rest."

Here is how my patient Barb, forty-four, head of her own public relations firm, learned to deal with emptiness. Barb, who was in treatment for overeating and excessive spending, grew up with three very lazy brothers. They never reached their educational or career potential, and, like their father, they struggled with varying degrees of alcoholism. Feeling great shame about their drinking and indolence, Barb was determined to be different—to achieve, be productive, and never waste time. She excelled in school and later built a fine reputation in her field while still very young. As she reached middle age, she began to experience symptoms of burnout.

Barb was tired and had to rest, but her attitude toward laziness interfered. She felt extremely uncomfortable just relaxing and couldn't tolerate unstructured time. She reported feeling empty and that her life had no meaning. To distract herself from such feelings, she started baking. Then she ate the cakes and cookies she produced and gained weight. Because she felt too anxious to stay home on Saturdays and enjoy a leisurely day doing nothing, she often went shopping for clothes she didn't need.

I shared with her that the emptiness and lack of meaning she experienced are part of the fabric of life. She needed to focus on those feelings, stay with them, and see where they took her—rather than try to numb them by cooking, eating, and buying. It was difficult for her to do, and many times she relapsed into her old habits. But as she gradually learned to accept her feelings, they were transformed and led her in a new direction.

She began to think about how tired she was of the business world, and she found herself reevaluating her career and her life. Never married, she realized that she really loved meeting new people outside of professional settings. She wanted to use her considerable people skills not to negotiate deals but to enjoy people. She had always dreamed of owning a bed-and-breakfast someday, and for the first time, she seriously considered it. Barb discovered that embracing feelings of emptiness, rather than dodging them, isn't the same as wasting time or being lazy. It can, in fact, lead to new insights and opportunities. Within two years, Barb sold her company and bought a small inn in the country. She's never been happier.

EATING ENOUGH

Another cause of emotional eating is not eating enough or restrained eating. The best defense against overeating is to eat. You may think, "I'll just eat a low-calorie breakfast and try to skip lunch." But by 3 P.M. you're hungry. Although you try to distract yourself, you're starving by dinnertime. By the end of the evening, you might consume 1,500 calories.

The decision to diet or skip meals is usually made as an attempt to improve appearance and enhance health and well-being. The cultural message since the seventies is that the solution to being overweight is to restrain eating and follow weight-loss diets. It has become clear that this solution has not resolved the problem. In fact, obesity has increased in the Western world. For the last 25 years, Janet Polivy, Ph.D., and Peter Herman, Ph.D., researchers at the University of Toronto, have investigated the effects of chronic dieting on women attempting to lose weight. They found that:

1. Restrained eaters display a tendency toward excessive eating when the restrictions are lifted.

2. There is a heightened emotional responsiveness in restrained eaters. They often respond very intensely and are more irritable, have cognitive problems such as difficulty concentrating on tasks, and tend to be overly focused on food and eating.

The point is, people who restrict their eating will eventually binge.

TAKE CONTROL BY TUNING IN

I often tell patients the story about the Zen Master at a party who is approached by a woman who asks him, "What is Zen?" He replies, "Do you want the long answer or the short answer?" She says, "This is a party, so I want the short answer." He says, "Zen is about paying attention." She responds, "That doesn't explain it to me. What's the long answer?" He says, "Zen is about paying attention, paying attention, paying attention." To overcome overeating, it is crucial that you begin to pay attention— pay attention to when you are hungry, when you are full, and when you are tired. You must ask yourself, "Am I confusing my need for rest or self-care with the need for food? If I am feeling deprived of essentials such as food and sleep, am I trying to fill myself up with food to keep going?"

For long-term weight loss, it is essential to learn to listen to internal cues about hunger. When you think you're hungry, ask yourself, "Am I really physically hungry, or am I tired and/or frustrated?" If the answer is, "It's 1 P.M. and I haven't eaten lunch," then you're hungry, and it's important to eat. But if the answer is, "It's 1 P.M., and I just had lunch at noon," then you're not physically hungry. In that case, look at your watch and wait fifteen to twenty minutes. Say to yourself, "I can eat all I want then, but first I have to wait that time."

During the fifteen to twenty minutes, explore what's going on for you. The internal conversation might run something like, "It's okay if I have to wait. I know I'm not physically hungry because I just had lunch. Maybe I feel hunger because I don't want to do laundry now or I don't want to get my driver's license renewed today, but I have to. That's why I'm turning to food."

After the wait, if you say, "Okay, the time has passed. Now I'm going to binge," that's fine. But there is one catch—you have to put all the food you're going to binge out on the table.

Why? Because it makes you aware of what you're eating. Patients say it takes some of the fun away, and it makes them think. They'll ask, "How many cookies do I need?" If it's ten, they'll pull out ten. Then all of a sudden they're actually looking at the quantity of food they are about to eat and it startles them.

This exercise helps patients develop the capacity to delay gratification and self-regulate. Self-regulation is the capacity to handle uncomfortable experiences or feelings without turning to something outside yourself, such as food, alcohol, or drugs.

Another aid to self-regulation is to keep a food journal to track how hungry and full you feel before and after eating. At every meal—or when you snack in between—rate yourself on a scale of 1 to 10, with 1 being the equivalent of "I am very hungry, famished" and 10 signifying, "I am stuffed, so full it hurts." How hungry are you? Rate yourself at all your meals today and see how you do.

ESTABLISH FOOD BOUNDARIES

At the times when you are vulnerable to emotional eating, you can also set boundaries for food and limit the amount you eat—if you take steps to protect yourself in advance.

Women will typically describe preparing a meal this way: "As I cut up the vegetables I start to eat those. As the rolls come out of the oven I start to eat those." That's what I call boundary failure. Or they'll say, "I wake up, and I want a bowl of cereal. I start pouring the cereal. I pour a lot. I eat all the cereal. I think, 'Okay, I already ate too much cereal.' Then I go back and get another bowl of cereal."

I tell patients, "When you're in a nonstressful situation, and you're not hungry, practice boundaries. If cereal is a problem, take the cereal and pour it into a bowl. Estimate what you think is one serving and put it into a Baggie. Do that for the entire box of cereal. It's easy to do. Now fill the cereal box with Baggies. Every morning, use just one prepackaged serving. What you're doing is teaching yourself boundaries, which is really what portion control is all about."

If you're someone who often overeats cake, do the same thing. Bake the cake and put icing on it when you're not stressed-out or hungry, so you won't be tempted to sample it. Cut the cake into healthy-size portions. Put each portion in a plastic bag. Place the bags in the freezer. Each day take out one bag. This way you can have a piece of cake as dessert or a snack, but you already have a boundary on it. Contrast this with walking in after work exhausted and eating half of a cake.

Ask for a To-Go Container

Overeating can occur because you have trouble eating properly in restaurants. If you overeat a lot when you're out, try this boundary suggestion: Every time you go to a restaurant, automatically ask the waiter to bring a to-go bag. Leave the amount you want to eat on your plate (and make sure there's enough food), but immediately put the rest into the to-go container. Place the container on the floor—and enjoy your meal.

EAT IN A MINDFUL WAY

When my oldest daughter went to Greece for a few weeks as part of a high school study program, I read the background materials that had been sent home with her. One reminder said, "Remember that everything shuts down for lunch from 12:30 P.M. to 2:30 P.M." The message was: There's no such thing as a quick lunch in Greece. In contrast, in the United States there is no respect or importance placed on meals, and the idea is to just have something to eat and to get it down quick.

The myth in our culture is that going faster is always better, even for meals. Nothing could be further from the truth. Americans can benefit greatly by slowing down and copying Europeans' mindful approach to food.

Mindfulness involves putting the spotlight on whatever you happen to be doing, and focusing on it exclusively. When you eat mindfully, you don't grab a quick bite or interrupt meals to answer the phone, which devalues the importance of the food and shows no respect for your meals. Instead, you put a spotlight on your eating each time you sit down at the table. You simply eat without also reading, working, or watching TV.

To eat mindfully, you not only put aside time to eat but you also make some rules that say, "This is a sacred time." Promise yourself, "I'm going to enjoy the food and the conversation." Light a candle, turn off the answering machine, and just be aware of how the food smells, tastes, and sounds as you eat it. Listen to the crunch as you bite into a piece of cucumber or an apple. When your mind wanders, take a deep breath and come back to the present.

You can eat in a mindful way if you're truly aware of what

you're eating and aware of the people with whom you're eating. Start by focusing on mindful eating at one meal each day. It will not only relax you but it will also help you notice when you're hungry and when you're full, and it will aid your digestion.

If you live alone, take yourself seriously and put aside time to enjoy a meal. Take out your best china, pour sparkling water into a wineglass, and enjoy the taste and smells of the food in front of you. Many women say, "I take out the good china only when company comes." But it's important to value yourself and treat yourself as well as you would treat your company.

Eat mindfully and you're also less apt to find yourself in the kitchen an hour later looking for food because it never really registered that you ate earlier. If you just walk in after a day at work, make a sandwich and take it with you as you walk up the stairs munching potato chips, you feel that you never had your dinner even though you consumed the calories.

MEALS AS RITUALS OF TRANSITION

Many midlife women report overeating during transitions, such as coming home from work or preparing to go to bed at night. Food seems to symbolize and facilitate the shift from one state to another, and these women head right for the cupboard or refrigerator at such times. To change this pattern, it's important to develop rituals of transition.

In recent years I have created my own rituals of transition for myself and my family. After seeing clients each day, I used to arrive home to be greeted by my children, all of whom wanted my attention at once. As soon as I walked through the door, I heard, "Look what we did at school today." Or, "I need you to go to the drugstore to get construction paper." And I'd listen to them while frantically trying to make dinner. Feeling stressed, I would then pour myself a glass of wine and nibble on food as I responded to their needs. Realizing that I needed to find a way to slow down the pace for all of us, I developed this ritual of transition.

When I get home from work on a cold night, for example, I first go to the garage to get a piece of firewood and bring it into the house. Then I hug each of the kids, telling them that I'll listen to their news and what they need after I get dinner started. I light a fire, put on a jazz CD, and go upstairs to change out of my work clothes. Once I'm dressed comfortably, I return to the kitchen, light a great-smelling candle, and start to make dinner. Then I sit down and give the children my attention.

I follow this routine each day. The repetition of the same sequence of events signals to both the children and myself that we are shifting into the rhythm of home life and slowing down for the evening. A sacred space is created for the family by playing the same music and sharing the same meaningful activities such as lighting candles and talking about the day at dinner. We, like many families, are probably too busy. But we're now all trained to expect this relaxed transition each night. The family shifts out of its high-octane state, and I find that I am much calmer.

Can you adapt some of these ideas, or think of others that fit your individual lifestyle? Rituals of transition are powerful tools for change. For example, to ease the shift from wakefulness to sleep, you might listen to soft music or read a chapter of an inspirational book. When you create your own calm ambience, you're less apt to seek solace in food.

As my clients work on these aspects of overcoming emotional eating, their behavior and thinking shifts. They find that they don't want to eat a bag of potato chips because they don't want to put fat and empty calories into their bodies, not just because they want to maintain their weight. They discover that they really can begin to develop a more positive body image. It's hard work, but it happens in workshops and in my office every single day.

5

EXERCISE FOR STRENGTH AND POWER

This journey into strength is not just about sculpting the body but how we can use the pathway of our bodies as a way to mine the strength in ourselves. For when external and internal strength are blended, balanced . . . that union of flesh and spirit is magnificent, radiant, a cause to rejoice.

—Karen Andes,
A Woman's Book of Strength

When Barb Harris, editor-in-chief of *Shape* magazine asked me to develop and lead the psychology component of their Positive Body Image project, she didn't pick me for my peak fitness level. I was chosen because of the work I do as a psychologist. Yet physical activity is part of these workshops, which include a one-day hike for five or six hours. The destination might be a beautiful boulder or stream, where I sit and eat lunch with workshop participants, and then give a lecture. The first time I joined a hike, which was partially uphill, I was the least fit of any of the women in the group. Huffing and puffing, I was the last one to arrive at the boulder. And although I felt exhausted, I had to lead a group discussion.

I remember thinking, "These women are in my age group, yet the hike didn't wear them out. They didn't turn red or need to stop and rest." The realization motivated me to do something about my lack of stamina. I loved the hiking experience and the feeling of exhilaration when I finally reached the boulder. I loved being up so high, and looking out on a spectacular vista. I thought, "This is a whole other world. This is what people do for leisure. They hike to beautiful places, and feel wonderful when they arrive—and I'm missing out."

That was several years ago, and though I'm still not one of the first ones to reach our hiking destination, I'm far more fit than I was then. I no longer feel that I can barely finish, and I'm not short of breath. My body has grown stronger through regular exercise, effort, and perseverance, and I enjoy the hike so much more. As I've improved my body's performance, I've strengthened myself psychologically, as well. I've gained confidence and developed leadership abilities, in my field and in other parts of my life, that I never knew I had.

With practice, your body can grow stronger and more competent, too, no matter what shape you're in now, no matter what your age—whether you're forty-four or sixty-four. To make it happen, however, you need to think differently about your ability to really change your body. You also need to redefine what you mean by a "good body." Is it one that sports a flat stomach or weighs 110 pounds? Although most women take that narrow view, I challenge you to move to a much broader definition. A good body is a strong, effective body. Body image is not just about how your body looks but also how it functions. Your own body ideal should include a standard of fitness.

Fitness is a critical goal because it maximizes your physical, intellectual, emotional, and social abilities, which makes you a more effective person. Effectiveness is the foundation of personal motivation and action, and we often think in terms of being effective psychologically. But women rarely consider how equally important it is to be effective physically—and that needs to change.

In his book *Self Efficacy: The Exercise of Control*, social psychologist Albert Bandura talks about building a resilient, effective self. People who do so overcome obstacles through perseverance, effort, and a strong belief that they can achieve their goals. Bandura observes that life is full of impediments and inequalities. To succeed in spite of them, you need to develop an optimistic view of your efficacy.

A NEW ROLE FOR EXERCISE

Instead of viewing exercise mainly as a way to lose weight, as most women do, it's time for you to look at it as a pathway to competence, skill mastery, and expansion of the capacity to function. You can start measuring success not just by a number on a scale but also by an increase in your stamina and power. In the process, you're going to start feeling a whole lot better about yourself. Women who exercise for fitness tend to have a more positive body image than those who exercise only to slim down.

Although there are many good fitness programs available, I like the balanced approach developed by physiologist Michael Hewitt, Ph.D., Health and Healing Director at Canyon Ranch Health Resort. Realistic about your time limitations, as well as your body's needs at your age, it involves five components: cardiovascular fitness; muscle strength and endurance; flexibility; balance and agility; and body composition.

CARDIOVASCULAR FITNESS

Cardiovascular fitness is a must because heart disease is the number one killer of men and women in the United States. Aerobic exercise such as walking, riding a bicycle, or taking an aerobics class strengthens your heart by causing it to beat harder and faster in order to pump blood to your muscles. It can reduce your risk of developing heart disease, it lowers blood pressure, and it has many other health benefits.

For minimum basic benefits, engage in aerobic exercise at a challenging level three or more times a week for at least twenty minutes, advises Hewitt. What constitutes challenging? Take the talk test. If you can converse normally while on the treadmill, pick up the pace. If you can't speak at all, you're working too hard. You should be able to carry on a conversation, but only in short, clipped sentences.

For a higher level of fitness, exercise four or more times a week for forty to sixty minutes.

To prevent tedium and avoid overworking any muscle or joint group, cross-train. For example, ride a bike to get to a place for a nice hike, or walk to the community pool for a swim. Whatever activities you choose, the key is to gently challenge the body.

MUSCLE STRENGTH AND ENDURANCE

Strength training is critical as we get older, especially for women. Starting at around age thirty, we begin to lose lean body mass at a rate of about ten ounces per year, Hewitt explains. The cumulative impact on the body is tremendous. If you lose lean mass regularly, you lose strength, and your metabolic rate slows. As a result, body weight increases, while mobility and function decline. However, that process can be prevented and reversed with strength training.

Strength training stimulates the development of muscle and bone. It helps you trim down, firm up, gain body definition and shape, and can help prevent osteoporosis. It also boosts your metabolism, because the more muscle you have, the more calories you burn.

Training involves strengthening arm, leg, and trunk muscles by lifting and lowering weights to the point of fatigue. It doesn't matter whether you choose free weights, machines, body work such as pull-ups or push-ups, or resistance bands, as long as you challenge your body.

Train twice a week for the basic minimum benefit. In cardiovascular exercise, duration is of prime importance. In strength training, the amount of time you spend on it has little to do with its effectiveness. "What matters is the challenge you give to your muscles. Most people train for an hour because they work with a trainer who bills by the hour. But you can get a good workout on most of your muscle mass in fifteen to twenty minutes or less," says Hewitt.

For enhanced fitness, train three times a week—or ideally, every other day. A longer program, which may run forty-five minutes or so, allows you to work on the entire body.

If you're a beginner, follow professional guidance at a health club or from a private trainer. If that is not possible, a good book on strength training for women, such as *Strong Women Stay Young* by Miriam E. Nelson, Ph.D., with Sarah Wernick, Ph.D., can be helpful.

FLEXIBILITY

As we get older, risk of injury increases due to physiological changes in muscles, bones, and connective tissue, changes that reduce suppleness, flexibility, and durability. Stretch exercises help avoid injury and discomfort, and they are probably the easiest exercises to work on because a small amount of stretching done frequently can be as effective as—or even more effective than—an hour-long stretch class done occasionally, according to Hewitt.

Choose three or four stretches that are the most challenging— remember that the ones you like are the ones you're already good at—and do them before and after exercising, including walking or jogging.

BALANCE AND AGILITY

This is the most ignored component of overall fitness, yet it not only protects you from falls and fractures but it also builds confidence. "You can tell people's functional age from two blocks away by the way they carry themselves. Wonderful agility and good balance enhance your mobility. Loss of agility and balance, on the other hand, can create a vicious cycle where diminished ability translates into diminished confidence," says Hewitt.

When you were a child you had great balance and agility because you skipped, played, and climbed trees. Somewhere in adolescence, however, you were encouraged to act like an adult and you stopped playing. Our culture has also exchanged agility for efficiency. We don't go hiking; we use a stairclimber. We don't row a boat capable of tipping, we use a rowing machine. We don't ride a bicycle with no hands, we use a recumbent bike at a health club.

Fortunately, you can improve your balance and agility no matter what your age by simply practicing. Try tai chi, a centuries-old form of exercise and self-defense that uses simple, rhythmic movements or, if you find that too difficult, ai chi, which is tai chi performed in the water. Sports such as tennis and soccer are superb, and even bowling has a balance component. Dance, whether social or aerobic, jazz, tap, or ballet, is also excellent for balance, and it offers the added benefit of enhancing relationships and intimacy.

And then there is Hewitt's favorite exercise for balance, which takes no additional time out of your day. Just stand on one foot each morning and evening while you brush your teeth. If you lose your balance, simply put your foot down or touch the vanity. Gradually you'll find that you can stand unassisted longer and longer.

Yoga and Pilates, both systems of mental and physical conditioning to strengthen and stretch the body, are superb for balance, agility, and flexibility, and they also include a strength component. They need to be supplemented, however, with cardiovascular exercise.

Every tradition of exercise is, in essence, a discipline of balance. Each move is followed by its mirror opposite. Stretching backward is followed by stretching forward. Reaching out to the right is balanced by stretching to the left. Periods of intense activity are followed by rest. To maintain a healthy sense of balance in life it is necessary to get up and stretch and move at frequent intervals throughout the day.

BODY COMPOSITION

"There's an obsession with body composition in our culture, particularly as we reach middle age, and especially in women. Your shape and level of body fat, and to a lesser degree your weight, broadcast your fitness. It's presumed that if you're slim, you're in great shape, and if you're overweight, you're in poor shape. But body composition is only one of the five components of fitness. Lots of slender people are in terrible shape," says Hewitt. He makes no recommendations for body composition because it changes as a consequence of other exercise components. However, many women who fall into the normal weight range are underlean, that is, they have lost enough lean body mass to reduce their strength and depress their metabolic rate.

A professional assessment of body composition, using techniques such as skinfold measurements and underwater weighing, can determine where you stand, and where to invest your limited exercise time. For example, if you have great lean mass but modest cardiovascular fitness, you need to devote more time to aerobic exercise. It may be possible to arrange an assessment through the physical education department of a local university; if not, the department can refer you elsewhere. In some areas, spas connected to hospitals for rehabilitation services offer the assessment.

Check with your doctor before starting a fitness regimen. The American College of Sports Medicine recommends a medical exam and cardiac stress test for healthy women over fifty planning to do vigorous exercise.[1]

In many cases, medical problems needn't stop you from exercising, although certain activities may be prescribed and others prohibited. If you have osteoporosis, for example, you might be told to avoid abdominal crunches, which can apply excessive pressure to the trunk and neck. The gentle controlled motion of tai chi may be recommended to improve flexibility for arthritis sufferers.

STRATEGIES THAT WORK

Now that you know what it takes to get in shape, the task is to get started and then stay fit. That's difficult for most of us. Over 60 percent of American women don't engage in enough physical activity, and over 25 percent don't exercise at all, according to the American College of Sports Medicine. To avoid contributing to these statistics, you need to do something different. Following are six strategies that work.

EXPLORE THE KIND OF MOVEMENT YOU ENJOY

I encourage you to pay attention to the type of movement you enjoy because which aerobic or strength training activity you do matters less than the fact that you do it. You won't stick with something you don't like, so try out different options until you find something that works for you. Some women prefer structured movement—going to classes, being part of a group, following a leader. Others hate being told what to do and like unstructured individual activities such as brisk walking, biking, skiing, or using a stepper or treadmill. Some enjoy movement that inspires more expression of the self, such as dancing.

Walking is especially good for women because it's convenient, involves no equipment or expense, and can stimulate bone growth, as it's a weight-bearing exercise, unlike swimming or cycling. It can be done alone or with a partner, and it is easy on the body. "After forty, many of us find that joints don't tolerate jogging well," notes Michael Hewitt.

It's great if you can afford to go to a health club, which allows you to try a range of activities. If not, YWCAs offer facilities that you can use for a less hefty fee. Also, many communities, especially in the suburbs, have recreation centers where individuals can attend classes and work out at low cost.

FIND PLACES WHERE YOU FEEL COMFORTABLE

If you're interested in a health club, check out a few of them before you sign up. Each club has its own energy, attitude, and type of people it attracts. Patients have told me, "I joined a health club where they want to take my weight and measurements, and then they want to check them again in six weeks. I'm a big girl. I don't want to be controlled." Women want to be in charge of their fitness, and they should be. They want to be in classes where teachers are sensitive to different body types and ages and to the fact that not everyone can keep up with the class or tolerate a high aerobic pace. Women also like to see teachers of different ages and shapes. If everyone is twenty and looks anorexic, it's intimidating.

I always suggest visiting at least three health clubs and choosing the one that seems most comfortable. If you don't feel at home in the place, you won't show up regularly.

Sometimes women have to make a place comfortable for themselves. The late Mabel Fairbanks was inducted into The Women's Sports Foundation Hall of Fame as a coach at the 2001 Annual Salute to Women in Sports Award Dinner on October 15, 2001. She could not perform competitively as a figure skater in the 1940s because she was black. Eventually she broke through the barriers, and she coached many other figure skaters, such as Kristi Yamaguchi and Tai Babilonia.

One of Fairbanks's mentees accepted the award for her. In the mentee's acceptance speech, she recalled Mabel describing the obstacles she'd faced as a youngster. When she'd go out on a skating rink—the only African-American youngster there—parents would often order their children to get off the ice, telling them that they weren't going to be on the same rink with "a nigger."

At first it was Mabel who got off the ice. But she soon decided not to do that anymore. She said to herself, "Good, let them get off. I'll have the rink all to myself." Mabel's ability to reframe a negative situation is an example we can all learn from. The ice rink wasn't a comfortable place for Fairbanks, but she made it comfortable. And because of her courage we now have African-American women skating in the Olympics. She's a role model for all of us.

SET A GOAL

Cindy, a corporate human resources executive who is divorced, already walks four times a week for forty minutes. At sixty-four, she is five feet three inches tall and slender, but she lacks upper body strength. She's determined to change now that she has a new boyfriend who takes her canoeing in Minnesota. "He has returned me to the joy of life at age ten at summer camp. I like canoeing because you have these packs and you can just put everything in the boat. On a hike you have to carry it all. But I get tired when I'm paddling because I don't have good muscle development.

"Here's a man who owns his own canoe. He's paddling in the stream and tells me, 'It's okay if you don't want to work so hard. I'll keep going without you.' But I don't like that. I want to pull my own weight and paddle on both sides. I'm useless on my left side."

When midlife women exercise, they often focus exclusively on aerobic exercise, as Cindy did, and ignore other fitness components. For many women, there's something mysterious and scary about weights. Women don't understand them the way they understand a treadmill. "They're so jockish," is the way Cindy puts it.

Cindy has rejected the notion that women are supposed to be physically fragile and helpless and has consciously decided to increase her strength and flexibility. She started moving toward that goal when her aunt treated her to a few days at a spa. "I didn't know anything about weights, but I'd been saying 'I've got to do something.' A trainer assigned to me introduced me to strength training. Now I work with weights twice a week and do stretches," says Cindy.

As she becomes a more active canoe paddler, she'll reap other benefits, as well. Canoeing has a cardiovascular component, depending on how rapidly she paddles, and it's excellent for balance. Lifting the canoe on and off the car and portaging it (carrying it around rocks in the stream) has a strength component. Depending on how far she reaches with each stroke, there may be a flexibility component. And if she canoes long enough and often enough, the activity will help increase muscle mass.

What is your goal? Do you exercise at all now? If not, aim first for aerobic activity. Add strength training, then work in flexibility, balance, and agility. If you already exercise, what gaps do you need to fill in? Aim for all fitness components and for a higher level of fitness. Strength training, for example, does things for your body that nothing else will accomplish.

A magazine editor who has been strength training for three years feels that she looks better than ever—at sixty-two. "I've never worn tank tops. I always felt they were too bare and accented my flabby arms. Now I wear them all the time because I have more definition in my upper body, which makes these tops look great on me. My arms aren't skinny, but they're a lot firmer than they were. Working with weights has changed everything. Something's happened to my bustline and shoulders so that they fit together better somehow. It isn't a matter of losing weight. I keep seeing myself in these tank tops, looking trim, and it makes me feel so good."

Focus on improvement in small increments. First you walk half a mile without stopping, but soon you can do a mile and a half, and before long you're up to four miles. First you hold three-pound weights when you strength train, but months later you're doing arm curls with ten pounds. The key is to gradually increase the challenge.

Set an exercise goal you want to accomplish. A good goal should have three components. It should be

1. *specific and measurable.* For instance, you can't just say, "I want to be more fit." Instead, say, "I'll be more fit when I can walk four 15-minute miles four times a week. That's my goal." A good goal defines what you're striving for.

2. *time limited.* Answer the question, When do I want to achieve this goal? In six months? Six weeks?

3. *achievable.* Be realistic. You don't want to set yourself up for failure. If you've never done aerobic exercise, it is unrealistic to expect to do four 15-minute miles in a few weeks. Nothing is more motivating than success.

Have a reinforcement system to reward yourself as you complete each step along the way. For example, if your goal is to complete a strength training program twice a week for twenty minutes, buy yourself a great new CD after training for one month. After two months, treat yourself to perfume that you love.

MAKE TIME

Any physical exercise is better than none. If you're going to meet your goal, however, you have to be willing and able to make it a priority. The circle exercise shown here helps you identify the demands on your time and the percentage of each day you spend on various activities. The first circle on the left is pretty typical for a working woman. It shows eight hours devoted to the job; eight hours to sleep; four hours to carpooling, TV, helping with homework, and hanging out; two hours to housework; one hour to a spouse, and one hour for personal time, such as talking to friends or relatives or getting a manicure. The second circle below it revises the time allocation to reflect exercise as a priority.

If you're serious about getting stronger, use the two empty circles at the right to clarify the demands on your time and to redistribute your time. Ask yourself, "If I add two strength sessions a week, how long will it take to get to the gym? How long will the sessions last? How long will it take to get back to the office or to home?" Or, "If I fast-walk four times a week, how long will it take?" Now redistribute your time in the circle. Maybe reaching your goal means you have to work 90 minutes less on strength training days. If you can't reduce your work schedule, maybe you can go in to the office early on those days and leave early for the gym or aerobics class. Perhaps you can organize a car pool to free up some of your time for exercise. Maybe your husband or children can make dinner or relieve you of certain chores, such as laundry. Can you pick up Chinese carryout on the way home from working out, instead of cooking dinner yourself? I say to my clients all the time, "Come on. Let's get creative here. What can change?" You need to say that to yourself to make the time to reach your goal.

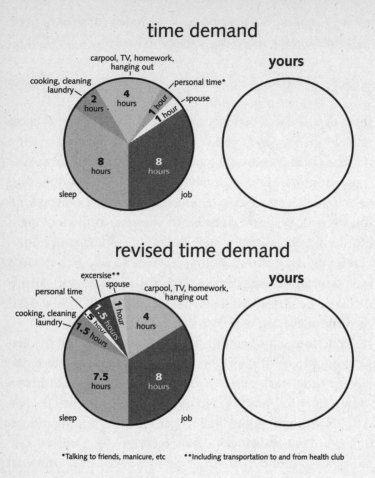

time demand

carpool, TV, homework, hanging out

cooking, cleaning laundry

yours

personal time*

spouse

2 hours 4 hours 1 hour 1 hour

8 hours 8 hours

sleep job

revised time demand

excersise**

personal time spouse

cooking, cleaning laundry

carpool, TV, homework, hanging out

yours

1.5 hours 1.5 hours 1.5 hours 1 hour 4 hours

7.5 hours 8 hours

sleep job

*Talking to friends, manicure, etc   **Including transportation to and from health club

THINK OF YOURSELF AS AN ATHLETE

The American Heritage Dictionary of the English Language defines an athlete as "a person possessing the natural or acquired traits, such as strength, agility, and endurance, that are necessary for physical exercise or sports, especially those performed in competitive contexts." Athletic women often focus on body competence and skill mastery and tend to have a more positive body image.

When I climbed that hill on my first hike, I kept saying, "I'm not real athletic. They didn't pick me because I'm fit." I made jokes about myself because I felt embarrassed about being the tail end of the hike. Since then, however, I've developed a completely different image of my body and what it can do. I've come to realize that joking "Oh, I never was an athlete" is the easy way out. Now I do think of myself as an athlete. I've acquired strength and endurance.

You can redefine yourself, too, even if you've never thought of yourself as an athlete, and even if you flunked physical education and were the last one picked for the volleyball team. Experience yourself as someone in training—not to be an Olympic star but to prevent osteoporosis, increase energy, handle other effects of menopause, and improve your body's performance.

Training is exciting for women—especially those who were overweight when they were younger and were badly mistreated—because they're not used to seeing themselves as athletes. One patient told me, "It's so much fun to tell people that I have a training schedule. They say, 'What! You're forty pounds overweight. Training for what?' I tell them that I'm training to hike part of the Appalachian trail." She also loves telling her grandchildren about what she's doing, acting as a role model for them, and showing them how much more energy she has, as she builds strength and benefits from cardiovascular exercise. What's more, she relishes regaining the energy she lost during menopause. Exercise actually energizes you.

You're Never Too Old to Compete

Abbie Britton Woods, forty-six and the founding editor of *Mode,* the first high-fashion magazine for women sizes 12 and larger, discovered training a few years ago. When she hit midlife, she realized that her metabolism and her body had changed. Always a runner and dancer, she loved moving. But after forty, everything she had ever done with her body plateaued. She couldn't maintain her shape.

Her solution was to try a competitive activity that would continually challenge her. She found a trainer who suggested a new sport: obstacle course competition. The course was a daunting one. She had to skitter up a thirty-five-foot cargo net like a squirrel and hurl herself over, then come down using only her hands. The next obstacle was a twelve-foot wall. She had to scale it with a rope and go over it, then go over a hurdle, followed by a balance beam. Then she had to pick up two forty-pound weights, sprint with them, vault over a fence, go under another fence, vault again, then negotiate a tire grid. And that was the short course.

Obstacle course competition was such a new sport that it was hard to find places to train. Abbie finally discovered an old course behind the Los Angeles Police Department Academy, which offered a wall, hurdles, and other equipment. "It was like splinter central, but my eleven-year-old son and I cleaned it up and it was perfectly good," she explains. After months of training, Abbie participated in the competition at age forty-four, ranking in the top ten among the competitors.

Now she competes on a much longer course, and she will soon teach a workshop on obstacle course competition called "Body Faith" in Burbank, California. Says Abbie, "When I started out, I thought, 'I don't have a lot of years left as an athlete,' but I was actually wrong. There is no age limitation. In one competition the most accomplished athletes were in their late thirties and forties, and most had children. Before I had my babies I always worried about gaining weight because I was a fat kid. When I was ten, I was five feet tall and weighed one hundred fifty pounds. Then I had my children and realized that if my body can do this, it can probably do anything."

Training and competing has also brought psychological rewards. Abbie has learned that because the body moves, action is more important in competition than thinking or talking—and that trying too hard can sabotage you. "Everyone has some kind of revelation about who they are in this course. You find out how you react in a situation where you meet obstacles. Overcoming them engages your fight or flight impulse because you have to think, 'Can I do this?'

For example, I stopped dead in front of the vaulting fence in the competition, but I beat the top time for the cargo net. Another woman got on top of the cargo net and started sobbing and couldn't get down. Everyone has a different response. The ones who do the course best are those who relax and let their bodies do the work. The winner of the competition did the entire thing with a smile on her face. But because I was new to it, I was aggressive, filled with adrenaline—and I fell off the balance beam, which is one of the easiest things. So you learn that less is more. You trust your body and your potential."

Abbie also discovered that everything she thought she'd be frightened of on the course was easy, and what she expected to be easy terrified her. "The obstacles I was afraid of were things that I thought about instead of acting upon intuitively. I realized that there was something about that which could be translated into life."

When you think of yourself as an athlete, your first obstacle may be getting up and walking to work instead of taking the bus. One of your goals might be participation in a new sport or a special event. Although few of us are ready, willing, or able to try an obstacle course like Abbie, you might realistically decide, "I want to join the five-mile Heart Marathon." Or "I want to kayak in Canada."

Be adventurous. Rafting and hiking holidays are available for beginners, as well as those at advanced fitness levels. They are wonderful ways to get out in nature and work on your body. Check out travel magazines and travel sections of newspapers for ideas. Inquire about local competitive events at health clubs and even large sporting goods stores, and ask athletic friends and neighbors for information.

After you've set the goal, research what is required to train for the activity. Go to the library and read about it. Check out resources on the internet. There may be classes you can take. Ask a trainer at the gym how to prepare. And remember, the qualities you develop in training will increase your chances of success in every facet of your life.

KEEP A JOURNAL

Many of us struggle with images of women as sex kittens in *Playboy*. We buy into the idea that we're objects who need to look a certain way to be accepted and loved—and we do whatever it takes. How can you reject such a path at age fifty-five? You move from thinking, "If I have a certain look, I'll be sexy and attractive," to becoming a woman who knows who she is and is sexy and attractive because of it. Exploring your physicality and feeling a sense of efficacy can help you feel confident about who you are. Writing in a journal is another way to develop a positive self-image.

In your journal, keep track of what you're doing each day to move toward your goal. If you want to walk for forty-five minutes four times a week, your entry might read, "I had to push myself out the door, but I walked for a half hour today. Only fifteen more minutes to go." If you plan to walk in a marathon, notice changes in your ability, such as: "Tuesday, Oct. 2. I have four more months before the marathon. I can walk four miles now without stopping. It's a slow rate, but I can do that. When I started, I could barely do a mile." Include details, such as, "Today it rained and I went on the treadmill since I couldn't walk outside."

Also explore feelings you're having about the exercise or about your body. One woman wrote, "I hate to leave the warm house to walk in cold weather, but once I get started, I'm amazed at how quickly I start sweating and peeling off layers of clothes. I feel such a sense of accomplishment when I'm finished that it doesn't matter what I do for the rest of the day. I've already achieved something." Expressing your feelings is important to help you shift your focus from, "How many calories did I burn?" to "I feel stronger and more competent after I walk."

I always tell women who want to train for a special event to remember the advice of Barbara Harris, editor-in-chief of *Shape* magazine: Keep a scrapbook in addition to your journal. Cut out pictures and articles about the event. Ask someone to take your picture when you cross the finish line. It's a way of cheerleading your own progress and declaring, "This is how I'm exploring my physicality in midlife."

Write down meaningful quotes by sports figures, such as this one by champion rock climber Lynn Hill: "Climbing not only teaches you the physical things that your body is capable of, but also the mental aspect."[2] Or clip quotes out of magazines and newspapers and use them in your journal and scrapbook.

WHAT'S GETTING IN YOUR WAY?

The strategies above do get you moving and keep you moving, but they won't do you any good if lurking psychological issues sabotage you. Women often succumb to these blocks to getting fit. How about you?

DISTORTED WAYS OF THINKING

Many women can't see themselves as athletic, a distortion that may have started when Mom said, "Don't run." Or, "You are so uncoordinated. You'll never be a cheerleader." Or when Dad sent the message that athletic women are unfeminine.

Journal writing led Abbie Britton Woods to childhood feelings that she had to hide her interest in athletics. In her family, which was highly intellectual, the attitude was "Athletes are stupid. Athletics are frivolous." When she made the decision to compete, she had to first face the message that it was bad to have the spotlight on her as a physical individual, and then she had to come out of hiding.

Another distortion may derive from fear of becoming too powerful. Pursuit of a strong, fit body can frighten some women who are afraid it will alienate others, especially men. I remember a midlife woman in one of my groups who said, "I love working out with weights, and now I can lift eight-pounders. But don't worry. I won't make myself into a powerhouse." Implicit in her statement was the message, "You're allowed to lift weights, but you don't want to get too strong. You don't want to intimidate any man." Young girls today may not feel this way, but I find it's a common attitude among baby boomer women I see.

Such distortions have to be confronted. Realize too that seeing yourself as an athlete doesn't mean that you have to be a body-builder or a soccer player. You can be someone who simply likes to put on sweatpants and run, or someone who gets out there to ski or swim.

SELF-CONSCIOUSNESS

Some women won't go to an aerobics or yoga class because they're afraid that they look fatter, older, or have more cellulite than other participants. Or they fear that they will be unable to perform the routines adequately and will look foolish. One woman who has dropped out of countless health clubs in the last twenty years explains, "I look so bad in my workout clothes. I hate being with women who look so much better than I do."

The fact is, you're getting too old to always compare yourself to others. It's important to develop an internal locus of control and react to the compass that is within you. Stop worrying about how you look. Build your sense of entitlement—that you have a right to be in this dance class, regardless of your weight and shape. Learn how to tolerate inequalities at the gym. The world is full of inequities. There will always be women in the room who are thinner or more athletic than you are. Don't let them throw you off balance. Focus solely on self-improvement. Think, "I was able to do aerobics for forty-five minutes straight, and a month ago I had to stop every twenty minutes to take a drink." Not, "Everyone else has better coordination than me." If you can stay focused on your own progress at the gym, you'll find that you can also focus on your own improvement in similar situations on the job—there will always be people who are more educated or more successful than you are—and elsewhere in your life. Keep the focus on you, rather than concentrate on comparisons with what others do or concern about what others will say.

Rhonda, who lives in New York City, tells the story of how she fast-walked on city streets. It bothered her that any time she'd reach a street corner and would have to wait for the traffic light to change, she'd have to step in place to keep up her heart rate. She felt that other pedestrians were wondering what was wrong with her. She happened to mention to her son that she felt embarrassed at these times, confessing, "I feel like an idiot."

Her son replied, "Mom, there are so many strange people on the streets, what makes you think anybody is paying attention to you?"

His retort changed Rhonda's whole perspective. "It made me realize how silly and self-centered I was. All these people were going about their business, thinking about their own lives, and I was sure they were all concentrating on me. It was a turning point. I stopped worrying about what strangers thought of me in other situations, too. It became, 'Who cares? I don't even know them.' "

BOREDOM OR LOSS OF MOTIVATION

Do you need to be courageous and try something different? Why not try kickboxing or tai chi or train for an event? Sometimes we are unmotivated because we've risen to a challenge, succeeded, and are now ready for another challenge.

In her book *Playing Like a Girl: Transforming Our Lives Through Team Sports*, author Marian Betancourt tells the story of a woman who joined a woman's soccer team in midlife. Among this woman's best moments "was early on [during the first year] when during a game I realized here I am at forty-five, and I can still learn a new sport and actually play and compete. The whole soccer experience has made me feel more like 'me.' " Betancourt writes, "She felt like the person she was in her teens, 'when the possibilities were endless and I felt powerful and effective and really liked the way I looked 'cause I was big and strong and in shape.' "

Helen, a financial planner who is single, took her first swing dancing class at age fifty-two. She told me, "Body-oriented stuff has always pulled me out of depression—yoga, massage, and now swing dancing. It's better than taking drugs! I feel so exhilarated.

"At home I look in the mirror and see someone who needs to lose fifteen pounds. When I'm dancing I look in the mirror and I don't look my age. I'm sweated up, my hair is flying, but I'm having fun—and it makes all the difference." She has also met new people in her class, including several younger men. That's not why she attends, but it's a nice bonus. The fact is, how we move affects how people perceive us, whether we seem energetic and fun to be with—or dowdy and depressed.

Helen dances three or four evenings a week, making it a key part of her nightlife. The activity helps her stay fit, too. "It's aerobic exercise," she points out. "You're constantly moving and bouncing up and down. Often you're waving your arms around. One piece of music leads into another seamlessly for twenty minutes at a time before you take a break. It's a wonderful workout."

OVERREACTION TO MISTAKES AND SETBACKS

When resilient people make a mistake, they don't beat themselves up. They turn missteps to advantage, using them as tools for growth rather than excuses for surrender. Failure is viewed as an informative experience that is part of the fabric of life, not a demoralization. When you fail, you get back on track, or you head somewhere new.

Marcy, a teacher and single parent of two children ages eight and ten, learned this lesson after participating in a binge eating group I led. Although Marcy, forty-seven, successfully stopped bingeing, she felt frustrated that she couldn't lose as much weight as she had expected. I suggested increasing her aerobic exercise and adding strength training to her workout. I also mentioned training for a fitness event, which would inspire her to exercise more frequently. A goal-oriented person, she immediately became excited about a leukemia bikathon slated for the following October. Marcy contacted a trainer, asked her to draw up a training schedule she could follow, and stuck to the regimen during the summer. Once school started, however, the demands on her time took their toll. With a full-time job and two sons to ferry to activities, she couldn't fit in training as well. Forced to drop participation in the bikathon, she felt disappointed and angry at herself for failing.

I encouraged Marcy to look at the setback differently. She needed to stand back and think objectively, analyze why she failed, and use the information to forge a new action plan. Pretty quickly she realized that her timing had set her up for failure. Fall was the busiest time of her year, and she had been unrealistic to expect to train intensively then. Spring and summer, however, would be ideal training seasons. She could limit her goal to an event scheduled for late July or August. And all the good feelings that would come from participating would carry her through the year.

GET COMFORTABLE BEING EFFECTIVE

It's not all downhill as you get older. I'm much fitter than I was when I was younger. There's no doubt that I've increased my cardiovascular capacity, because I now walk five days a week—and sometimes six if the weather permits and I'm not traveling too much—and cover four miles in an hour along a beautiful nature trail. I'm building stamina while experiencing the healing elements of nature. I've struggled with my strength and I'm really excited right now because I'm lifting ten pounds in arm curls. To me, that's a lot.

You can grow in physical strength, too. As you do, you're going to build mental strengths and develop more of a voice in the world. It's all part of what can be fabulous about midlife. You can discover "Wait a minute. I can lift my carry-on bag and stow it up there in the airplane compartment without anyone's help—at age sixty-two. When I was forty-five I had to wait for some man to come by and put it up there for me. I can play golf without a golf cart and walk the course; three years ago I couldn't. I can go to a wedding and dance all night."

Exploring fitness is valuable in and of itself. But it can also lead to a greater goal, such as personal growth, because everything you experience in your fitness program is symbolic of what goes on in life. For example, Maria, a Latina woman, saw parallels between working on her exercise regimen and working on her dissertation. Recently divorced, Maria went back to school for her Ph.D. at age fifty-two—and concurrently started exercising for the first time in her life. She observed that her dissertation and her fitness program both required long, hard work and had a distant finish line. In addition, success in both cases depended on perseverance and her ability to stay motivated and concentrate.

When you focus on fitness, you may also shed pounds. It's clear from research that exercise is really the most crucial component of weight loss because it affects metabolism and burns calories. In addition, it releases endorphins, which produce a natural high for people and decreases anxiety.

When your body is strong and effective you're going to experience yourself as healthy, sexy, and energetic. I find I always pay attention to women who feel that way about themselves, whether they're a size 8 or a size 16. So does everyone else.

6

COMMIT TO DELIBERATE SELF-CARE

It is never too late to be what you might have been.
—George Eliot,
The Quotable Woman

I learned a lot about what it means to tend your body well several years ago, just after I had my third child. I was an invited speaker on body image at a demanding conference at the University of Ghent in Belgium, which left me feeling totally exhausted. I was discussing the grueling pace with an American couple I met at the conference, when they happened to ask, "Have you ever been to the spa in Versailles, outside Paris? It overlooks the palace gardens and is a wonderful place to recharge and unwind."

No, I explained, I'd never been there and planned to go right home. But I felt so tired that I suddenly decided, "You know what, I'm going to take the train to Paris to stay at this place." Because it was August and the French were all on vacation elsewhere that month, the rates were low. I called my husband to tell him, "I'm staying here three extra days because I'm really worn out." He wasn't happy about this change in plans, but I knew that I had to do it for myself.

In spas in the United States, the food is low fat, low calorie, and women participate in constant exercise activities to get in shape.

This spa was different. Arriving hyped-up from the conference, I checked into my room. Then I walked over to see the person who organizes your personal schedule. "I want to do everything here," I told her. "I just came from Belgium, and I've never been to a spa in Europe." She immediately replied, "I think you need to sit outside awhile. We're going to talk there. I'll get you a glass of wine, and you can relax and look at the gardens and the animals." The animals were sheep grazing within this magical, serene setting.

When the woman returned, she said, "I don't think you should try so many activities. We actually have very few classes. What we do have is long delicious meals, wonderful massages, and skin treatments."

This spa was not about losing weight—it was about taking loving care of yourself. Women walked around in robes, rather than aerobic outfits. Three-course meals included wine. After lunch, I'd fall asleep in a state of total relaxation. Instead of scheduling an activity every hour, I went with the flow of the day.

Because I'd never had a skin treatment before, I looked forward to it. And it was perfectly tailored to my needs as a woman who recently gave birth. The clinician said, "Oh, you had a baby. Your skin is probably dry and needs nourishment." She also said, "You've got that belly that women have after they've carried a baby. Let us massage it with special oils."

In the United States, masseurs don't touch your breasts or belly. They do your back, your legs, and arms. But the French, who don't think twice about going topless at the beach, are more comfortable with the body—all of it. I had a massage the day of my skin treatment, and it felt marvelous to have my entire body tended to. As she worked, the masseuse spoke to what was human in me. "Aren't our bodies amazing?" she asked. "Can you believe that six months ago your baby was inside of you?"

I was also advised not to turn on the TV in my room. "Most of the stations are not in English anyway. Just lounge by the fireplace, read, and relax," said the woman in charge of my schedule. "Instead of running around, walk over to the palace of Versailles." She added information on the best times to avoid the crowds and urged me to attend a gala party scheduled at the palace for a French holiday. "People from the press will be there. Just arrive as if you're a reporter, and have fun," she instructed.

Unprepared for a formal evening at the palace, I of course had nothing to wear. Normally I'd think, "I'm taking three extra days to be here and it's costing more money. I shouldn't dare buy a long dress." But I felt so entitled that I went shopping, finding just the right style at a local boutique. On a beautiful night, I walked to this formal party at the palace of Versailles—and I felt like a million bucks.

For me, the spa experience was a great example of moving out of my cage. I relish the memories, which have taught me so much. The relaxing pace gave me time to get back in touch with myself, not as a mother or wife or psychologist, but as a woman. I'd had no time to myself since the baby arrived. I had been so busy that I didn't feel sexual. The solitude helped me center myself. Often we think "I'll lose this weight (or "I'll have a tummy tuck") and then I'll feel sexy and like a woman again." For some that approach works. For me, however, it was this retreat, which had never been an option before, that provided a sense of renewal. When I got back home, I felt revitalized. I couldn't wait to see my husband and children again.

European women of all ages feel entitled to take care of their bodies. For them, it's an essential part of being a woman, and a natural part of their elegance. Beauty salons in France routinely offer a buffet of body care services because women, including older women, expect them. There's an "Institute of Beauty" on every other street specializing in skin care and other beauty essentials. Most American women are never taught to feel that their bodies are worthy of such tender treatment. Following the example of French women can do wonders for our body image and self-esteem.

Do you feel entitled and act like it? A male patient I worked with early in my career did. I was at my first job in the psychiatry department of the University of Cincinnati, where I treated a lot of women who had to lose weight for health reasons. When they couldn't do it, they were referred to me by cardiologists and other physicians. They'd walk in and say, "My physician says I have to lose weight. I just had a heart attack. I was in intensive care. What's wrong with me? I can't seem to follow the diet I was given." The diets were 1,200 or 1,500 calories.

Then one day a cardiologist referred a man. He sat in my office on the edge of the couch, holding a paper—which turned out to be his diet. Almost throwing it at me, he exclaimed, "You know something is wrong with a doctor who asks a man as busy as I am to eat eighteen hundred calories a day. Doesn't he realize that I'm up at 6 A.M. I work all day; I get home at 6 P.M.; I help my wife with the kids; I go to bed at 11 P.M. Eighteen hundred calories a day is not enough gas for my car."

I've always remembered that experience as a fascinating example of how men feel entitled and women don't. Instead of assuming, "Something's wrong with me," men say, "Something's wrong with the doctor." They feel entitled. When I tell this story to a woman, she'll respond, "I'm a busy woman, too. I have three children. But I'd never dream of questioning the doctor about whether the diet allows enough food for me." She just assumes the problem is that she's out of control.

Isn't it time that attitude changed? The way you do or don't take care of yourself reflects your body image. If you value your physical self, you treat it lovingly, paying attention and listening to what you need and daring to go for it, in addition to setting healthy weight goals and exercising. The body is like a computer; it can't help what's programmed into it at age ten. But you can redirect that program now and make self-care a priority in your life.

DEVELOP A DELIBERATE ATTITUDE

One of the building blocks of change involves deliberately setting out to be different. In a book entitled *The Resilient Self*,[1] researchers studied the effects of parents' mental illness on their children's adjustment. Although it was initially assumed that a high percentage of youngsters whose parents were alcoholic would themselves become alcoholic, a majority of the children did not.

The researchers went on to study the 75 percent of children who did not become alcoholic, and they described the deliberate attitude these resilient youngsters adopted. They observed their parents' lifestyle and then decided to improve upon it. They married into strong, healthy families and developed meaningful family rituals. They seemed to repair themselves by actively deciding to live differently from their parents, making healthy choices to strengthen themselves and to battle the adversity within. Instead of coming home and drinking at night as their parents did, they scheduled leisure activities or coached their children's sports teams.

It takes this same kind of attitude to improve a negative body image. Change involves understanding the past, and applying that knowledge to make life better. Usually there must be a conscious, and at first often psychologically uncomfortable, shift in behavior. Many people feel selfish or guilty about taking care of themselves. It is hard work, and it must be deliberately undertaken. For instance, change requires you to acknowledge your limitations instead of trying to make your body perfect, and to employ a number of active strategies. Following are five strategies to encourage more self-care in your life. Each is to be practiced each day.

ADOPT CARING BEHAVIORS DAILY

Engaging in activities every day to comfort, soothe, relax, pamper, and strengthen your body will help you create a lifestyle that supports and insists on acceptance of your body.

There are so many ways to be good to every part of you. You can take bubble baths, treat yourself to a massage, or find a nurturing hairdresser who gently shampoos your hair and creatively styles it. Find clothes that express who you are right now in your life and are comfortable enough to make you feel relaxed. Finally, instead of exhausting yourself, appreciate the value of rest by discovering the art of napping.

RATE YOURSELF

One of the tools that can help you start treating your body like a worthy asset is a rating chart that you fill in each day. Take a piece of paper and write down a goal, such as "I am going to accept my body and take care of it." To see how close you are getting to this belief, score yourself on the chart from 0 to 100 percent. The first day you might be only 20 percent of the way toward believing that statement. But gradually you might creep up to a score of 50 percent, which means you're halfway to accepting your body and taking care of it. As you score yourself each day, the idea is to see how much closer you are to firmly holding that belief.

KEEP A DAILY ACTIVITY LOG

To improve your rating, record observations about yourself that are consistent with a more positive body image. Start a daily activity log in which you notice and record moments when you feel accepting and good about your body. This is difficult because the assignment asks you to look for or perceive experiences that you may naturally tend to ignore or distort. To help identify them, think of areas where positives are possible, as illustrated in the following entries:

> "I brushed my hair for five full minutes and it felt so soft and shiny."

> "I taught my husband how to touch my body in a more nurturing way."

> "I bought a form-fitting dress that made me feel sexy."

> "I turned off the TV when a comedian made fun of fat women."

> "I used a creamy lotion on my dry legs. Instead of itching, they felt nourished, sleek, and smooth."

> "I loved wearing a new cologne at my wrists, behind my ears, and at the bend in my elbows."

> "I looked in the mirror this morning and thought, 'You look so good today.' "

People think that body image is about weight and shape, but in fact, body image can change based on what you do each day and how your body functions. It's important to widen your definition to include more than just your appearance. We know from research that if women eat healthy all day, for example, they feel better about their bodies even though they've got the same body they had yesterday. Remember to include in your log behaviors that made you feel good, such as, "I got up and danced at the party. What fun!" Or, "I moved up to eight-pound weights today. It was tougher, but I did it." Or, "I wore my favorite blue velour pants. The fabric feels so good and comfortable."

Begin also to note times when you pay attention to feeling tired and then rest, or recognize that you're hungry and then eat. Patients find that as they increase such behaviors, their body acceptance scores rise on the rating chart.

As you keep track of self-care activities every day, you will expand your awareness to notice good feelings, such as, "I feel more energetic than ever." Gradually you can begin to accept your body as a positive source of feelings, physical needs, and information about yourself. Then when you feel stressed or bad, you can realize that there are other actions besides bingeing that you can take to feel in charge and in control. For example, if you're upset over a fight with your sister or husband, you can work out for an hour instead of filling up on chocolate layer cake. Or you can discover other options, such as taking the kids ice-skating. Start a self-care cupboard at home, filling it with items you can turn to when you need them. They might include the phone number of a supportive friend you can call when you feel sad, books or poems or affirmations that inspire you, and wonderful CDs that feed your soul.

VISUALIZE

Every night before you go to bed, close your eyes and picture yourself engaging in positive body behaviors the next day. Include details, to paint as rich a picture as possible. For example, visualize a situation where you're attending a conference. A colleague wants to meet you for a drink before dinner, but you want to swim in the hotel pool before dinner. Imagine yourself warmly and confidently telling your colleague that you can't have a drink before dinner, but you do want to sit next to her at dinner to catch up. Then see yourself swimming in the pool. Visualize yourself accomplishing your goals step by step and overcoming obstacles.

In her data log, a compulsive overeater named Sharon described waking up feeling depressed. She wrote, "I looked in the mirror, and felt disgusted at how fat I was. I wanted to stay in bed all day and order pizza." However, because she had been working on her log the night before, she remembered action strategies that she could use to feel better. She got up, took a walk, and then put on her favorite dress. She described feeling better about her body as the day went on.

REALIZE HOW YOUR MISTREATED BODY FEELS

I use the following exercise to help women understand what their bodies go through when they mistreat them. I ask them to name the body area that dissatisfies them most. Then I direct them to pretend to be that part, such as thighs or hips, and write down the answers to the questions below on a sheet of paper:

1. What is it like to be a body part in Sally's body?
2. How does Sally treat me?
3. What would I want to tell Sally? What do I need from her at this point in my life?

One woman who dislikes her belly wrote, "My stomach told me, 'Listen, I have held three of your children and they are one of the joys of your life. You've been divorced, but you have a great relationship with your children and their life started inside of me. I'm getting tired of being criticized and put down. You can't have the stomach you used to have, but without your stomach now, you wouldn't have those children either.' I never looked at it this way before."

Another stomach complained, "All of this obsessing and dieting is hurting me. You are making me ache because you don't eat much all day. I get so hungry. Then you put so much in me at night. And you're always so negative about me. I want to be taken care of better."

Someone unhappy with her flabby arms wrote, "My arms said, 'I have held and carried everything you need all your life. I've never failed you when backpacking, carrying your briefcase, or lugging grocery bags into the house. I'm sick of you worrying about how I look. The only thing I want you to do is strengthen me some.' "

Another woman who suffers from body hatred wrote, "My body said, 'You are like a slum landlord because you neglect me. You don't take care of me and then you have the nerve to hate me and complain about me. You aren't consistent. For a few months you eat healthy, but then you give up and eat crazy. When you're frustrated you put all these potato chips and diet sodas in me. It makes me sick. You don't pay attention to when I'm hungry, and I growl. You don't pay attention to when I'm full. I'm getting older and I'm getting tired of this.' "

Participants tell me that this exercise helps target ways to be more loving and kind to their bodies. Challenge your own thinking and try it yourself. Decide which part of your body bothers you most. Pretend to be that part. Then answer the questions on your own sheet of paper. Develop an action plan based on your answers. Remember, awareness is the first step in change.

REDUCE STRESS

Part of self-care involves relaxation and stress reduction. Exercise in general is a wonderful stress reducer. Do it daily. It elevates your mood and shifts your focus from your troubles to experiencing your body. Yoga and tai chi are particularly excellent for this.

Make the time you set aside to exercise a time of renewal and caring for your needs. Tape an interesting movie or TV program and watch it while you're on the treadmill at home. Listen to a motivational tape while you're on the stepper. Take your child on a walk outdoors, where you can appreciate and notice nature together, enjoying an intimate, enriching experience. Feel the sense of community as you move in an aerobics class with other women.

Set aside twenty minutes each day to relax, too. Relaxation is vital to countering the stresses in the body caused by your nervous system's fight or flight response. You can write in a journal, listen to music, meditate, read poetry, or simply find a comfortable chair, put your feet up, and let your mind meander.

EDUCATE YOURSELF ABOUT MENOPAUSE

Part of taking care of yourself involves being well informed about menopause and its effects on your body. Menopause, which is diagnosed when menstruation has ceased for twelve months, usually occurs somewhere between the ages of forty and fifty-five. In the United States, the average age is fifty-one, according to the American College of Obstetricians and Gynecologists. Menopausal symptoms, such as hot flashes, can cause discomfort and may impact on some women's quality of life. However, today there are effective ways to manage these symptoms.

For example, I experienced bleeding in the middle of my menstrual cycle, which often occurs in perimenopause, the period surrounding onset of menopause. Since such breakthrough bleeding can be a sign of a malignancy, my doctor performed a biopsy. When the results were negative, he advised me to take birth control pills, which regulate the menstrual cycle. But I resisted the idea, wary of possible side effects, such as blood clots, and feeling that I was too old to take the pill. A year later, however, the bleeding suddenly went out of control. It was frightening. There was so much blood I thought I was having a miscarriage.

I had another biopsy, and again my doctor said, "You're fine, but you really should go on the pill." Although I still didn't like that idea, my resistance waned as the heavy bleeding continued and began to have ramifications.

I never knew when it would start. I was light-headed and irritable. I was beginning to feel nonsexual. I was also about to go on a family vacation at the beach. I love to swim and play volleyball with the family, but I realized that I couldn't even wear a bathing suit. I'd have to wear shorts. I thought, "This is perimenopause— you're stuck with it." I felt trapped.

Realizing that I couldn't go on this way, I read up on the pros and cons of the pill, and questioned my doctor further. I decided that I had to try the pill. Once I started, the bleeding stopped right away. I felt great. It was so freeing, and it taught me how important it is to check out your options. If you don't do your homework, you can really suffer needlessly. Now I've got my life back.

Perimenopause and menopause do cause changes. Fluctuating estrogen levels in perimenopause may result in hot flashes, mood swings, fatigue, insomnia, and other symptoms. Estrogen levels continue to drop in and after menopause, causing vaginal dryness and loss of elasticity as vaginal tissue thins or dries out. For some women, sex becomes painful. Fortunately, there is help available. Vaginal lubricants and estrogen vaginal creams can help keep sex pleasurable. Hormone replacement therapy (HRT), which consists of estrogen plus progestin, can banish hot flashes and relieve certain other menopausal symptoms, as well as help reduce the risk of osteoporosis. However, HRT is also associated with increased risk for breast cancer and other conditions. It's a complicated decision and an individual one that you should make with your health care provider.

Menopause is a natural process. Like most transitions, it involves losses and gains, as well as a cycle of growth and change. Most women do not experience severe symptoms that interfere with their lives. And what people rarely talk about is that right after the transition, postmenopausal women report feeling better than ever.

NOURISH YOUR SPIRITUALITY

One of the psychological tasks of midlife is to tap into your spirituality. It's a time to be deliberate about listening to the soul within you and nourishing yourself through an organized religion, the arts, nature, or reading about spiritual teachings. Connecting to your inner self is essential for a positive body image.

My mother, who found comfort in her religion and was a very spiritual woman, taught me that the body is simply the house you live in. She said that the life force in you, the essence of who you are when shorn of the trappings of your many roles in life, is your spirit. When I was a teenager, I found that there was little to rebel against in my mother. She wasn't very controlling because she had liberal political beliefs and was interested in the women's movement. As my statement of individuation, I therefore rejected religion and the importance of spirituality in my life. But not for long. As an undergraduate, I became involved in a dance project, where I often felt spiritually transformed through movement, improvisation, and choreography. I took a class on meditation, which is a process of contemplation and reflection wherein the goal is a state of relaxed but alert awareness. I began to meditate on a daily basis. During graduate school I found myself drawn to books and workshops exploring the connection between spirituality and psychotherapy. When I began to practice psychotherapy, I used movement, music, candles, and the same incense that I smelled in church as a child to develop therapeutic rituals to help women overcome shame and loss.

As I became increasingly involved with work and my family, the days I meditated became few. In my personal life I could not ignore the miracles of pregnancy and childbirth, and the often difficult but transpersonal aspects of being a parent, a close friend, and a partner. But my spiritual practice lacked in consistency. When my mother died, one of the gifts her loss brought was a reminder of the importance of spirituality. Her death reminded me that I had to be deliberate about cultivating my spiritual self.

One way to cultivate spirituality in your life is through meditation, which is really about taking the time to experience your own core. To meditate, you have to sit, be still, and empty your mind of distracting thoughts. There are several kinds of meditation; for example, you might focus on your breath or on a mantra, which is a word or words that you choose and repeat over and over again. You can meditate anywhere. I try to devote twenty minutes to it every day. Sometimes it is a very relaxing and even a mystical experience. Other times I have difficulty slowing down and experience many distracting thoughts. I have to remind myself that the practice of meditation isn't about perfection. It's about always coming back to your breath and knowing that distracting thoughts are part of the process. Just as in life, when you get off the path, the key is to just get back on.

The cumulative effect of meditation over time has been very positive for me, and research confirms the beneficial effect of meditation on the mind and body. It helps reduce tension and anxiety, and alters our mental state. Make room in your schedule to be quiet, to meditate and listen to the wisdom of a still body.

Meditation is actually a Buddhist spiritual practice. Buddhism also teaches to live in a mindful way. The practice of mindfulness, which is attentive, heedful awareness, helps you gain insight into your reactions, perceptions, and behaviors, and it helps you handle stress in daily life.

When I'm with my children, for example, I try to put the spotlight on them and stay focused on them, not the phone or my mental to-do list. When I'm eating, I might try to really focus on the texture and smell of the food, not get lost in a TV program.

The more mindful we are of the present moment, the more we allow ourselves to really be there—and the less stress we experience. In his book *Timeshifting*, Stephan Rechtschaffen calls stress our resistance to the present moment.

My eight-year-old son taught me a lesson about being in the present moment last December when he went Christmas shopping with me and my mother-in-law, who has Alzheimer's. As the three of us approached the mall, I began to feel stressed about my extensive shopping list: a football for my older son, Michael, a manicure set for my eldest daughter, Kristin, and twin baby dolls for her younger sister, Jennifer. Jonathan said that he couldn't wait to buy his presents and then, with his own money, stop off for ice cream.

Granmom, who wasn't talking, but smiling, and walking along with us, stopped suddenly. Although Jonathan and I encouraged her to keep walking, she stood still. I tried to reassure her that we would walk with her, but she looked back at us with blank eyes.

Jonathan said, "Mom, what are we going to do?"

I didn't know the answer, and I grew anxious thinking, "How can I get my mother-in-law to walk? Will I be able to buy the presents today? If not, when?"

Suddenly, Jonathan turned, and in a loving way said, "Grandma, watch me. Take baby steps like me." And she began to move—one baby step at a time. I began to walk in baby steps, too. We moved slowly through the mall. I saw the sparkle in Jonathan's eyes as he led his grandmother. Approaching the ice cream stand, he told me,

"I probably shouldn't buy the ice cream because if Grandma stops it might take a long time to get her moving again." I agreed with him. He acknowledged that it would be hard for him to give up the ice cream, but he would keep walking.

I took a lesson from Jonathan and stopped resisting the moment. I gave up on my list of presents to buy—and experienced the beauty of Jonathan's glow as he held his grandmother's hand and she smiled back at him.

Do you overcommit and resist the moment, angry and frustrated because you are forced to wait in line at the supermarket or at the bank? Can you accept the waiting, calm your body, and allow yourself to listen to the music being piped through the store? Can you use it as a time to imagine a beautiful celebration coming up with family and friends or a wonderful vacation?

You can learn to tolerate feelings of ambivalence, engage yourself in affirmation, and experience the joy in each situation by practicing meditation and mindfulness. When these behaviors become part of your daily life, your body image improves. Research shows that when people prepare for a fitness event, eat well, and use relaxation methods, such as meditation and mindfulness, they tend to feel good about their bodies.

Tremendous changes have taken place in our lives. The world is exhilarating, yet exhausting, frightening, and lonely at times. Let's make sure that we build into our daily lives time to stop and listen to our inner voices.

You can't be fully alive unless you are able to acknowledge and access your spirit. Let your spirit radiate from you. It's one of the unique and attractive aspects of your persona.

TEACH OTHERS HOW TO TREAT
AND TALK ABOUT YOUR BODY

In a national survey I conducted with Ruth Striegel-Moore, Ph.D., on body image for *Psychology Today,* I asked women, "Who are the people who have affected your body image?" I expected the answers to predominantly list people from the past, but to my surprise those from the present played an equally important role. Are there people in your life now who are critical of your appearance—your spouse, boyfriend, child, parent, sibling, or coworker? Regardless of who they are, you can let others know that you won't tolerate hurtful comments about your body.

One way to handle criticism of your appearance is to use your voice to tell them what you do want—as a woman in one of my workshops did. She'd come home every night and say to her husband, "Oh my pants are so tight. I can hardly button them." He would reply, "If you'd eat less, they wouldn't be so tight." She taught him to behave differently. "When I come home tired and I berate my body," she instructed, "I want you to say nice things and give compliments instead of agreeing with me." He heard her, and he followed her instructions.

Another strategy is what I call the Roseanne Response, which I've named after the client who shared it with me. When people made intrusive, negative remarks about her body, she employed a simple yet effective comeback. If someone said, "It looks like you gained weight," she would say bemusedly, "And you are saying this because? . . ." By questioning the purpose of the comment, she shifted the burden of explanation back to the critical person, where it belonged. Over time, such remarks virtually ceased. Her response helped her experience power in a new way. She no longer felt that she had to change her body. She could refuse to accept others' definitions of how she should look. She stopped reacting to criticism and began living.

If someone comments on what or how much you eat, reply, "You may eat what you want, but I am eating this." What if someone replies to a Roseanne Response with "Oh, I was worried about you"? Answer quite directly, "You can help me by walking with me at lunchtime rather than by commenting on my weight." It's empowering to realize that you don't have to put up with cracks about your body or behavior.

ELLEN'S STORY

Ellen went to the doctor for a checkup. Concerned about her health, he told her, "You have mitral valve prolapse, high cholesterol, and you're starting to put on a lot of weight. I'd go to a nutritionist and try to get some exercise to see if you can make some improvements."

Taking his good advice, she started walking five times a week, did strength training twice a week, and made better food choices. When she returned to the doctor a year later, he exclaimed, "Wow, you look great. Your cholesterol is in the normal range, and you've lost six pounds and kept it off." She assured him that she felt more energetic, too, and was even starting to hike regularly. "Whatever you're doing, keep it up," he told her.

At home that night, she looked in the mirror and mused to herself, "He was right. I do look great. I may be a little curvier than most, but it looks good." Just at that moment, her husband walked in. "What are you doing?" he asked. She told him about her visit to the doctor and his enthusiastic response to her progress. "But what did he say about that forty-six-year-old ass?" he retorted.

She fired right back, "Well, he was busy. We didn't have time to talk about you today."

Sometimes people feel uncomfortable when you accept your body. But that doesn't mean you have to allow them to make negative comments about you. Taking care of herself was a growth experience for Ellen. She had become stronger in mind as well as body. She wasn't going to tolerate insults and put-downs. Her husband said an awful thing to her, but her comeback put him in his place.

In your daily log, keep track of the ways you react to feedback about your appearance. Refuse to play the role of victim, and take charge. Define yourself and your body image by what you do each day, not by how others respond to you.

We all have choices, and we must be deliberate about creating a lifestyle which increases the odds that we will feel good about our bodies. Cultivate relationships with people who are comfortable with their own bodies and who routinely flatter each other with compliments. They will provide a positive environment for body acceptance.

DEAL WITH SABOTAGE

A workshop participant made up her mind to lose twenty pounds. She went to Weight Watchers and began working out. While on her treadmill at home one evening, she overheard her fifteen-year-old daughter complain to her father, "Now that Mom's trying to lose weight, she only thinks about herself. She's always exercising."

I often hear similar stories from women in the groups I lead. Someone will say, "I finally did it. I got serious about eating healthy and exercising, and look what happens." And yes, it does happen. In an ideal world family members and others who love you would say, "I'm so glad that you're taking your health more seriously." But that's not the way life always operates. Others sometimes have negative reactions during your process of transformation.

Losing weight and getting fit can shake up your relationships.

You change when you commit to taking charge of your body. You're less available timewise, and your focus changes. Since you don't operate in a vacuum, your success leads to shifts in other parts of your life, as well. You take better care of yourself and take yourself more seriously. For some people, a more confident, powerful you is a scary change, which they unconsciously try to stop. Enter diet sabotage.

Diet sabotage frequently comes from your husband or boyfriend. Although initially he might have been happy that you wanted to lose weight and was supportive of your effort, he might have assumed that you'd only do this for a few weeks. His attitude might have changed after you started making progress and it became clear that you were going to continue. He is not prepared for the kinds of changes that occur when you're committed to achieving and maintaining a realistic goal weight.

Like your children, he may resent that you're out walking every day or going to the health club. He misses the snacks you used to share every night. He resents attending the kids' games by himself because you're working out. He may even worry that you are now interested in attracting other men—or that you'll try to get him to lose weight as your next project. On the other hand, don't go overboard yourself. Keep balance in your life.

DEFENDING AGAINST SABOTAGE

You get positive feelings from sticking to your health plan, but you may also face negative feedback from others, which you need to confront and deal with. To combat negative feedback, establish that you really want to stick to this health plan, and have the courage to do it. Then use inner applause to support yourself. Tell yourself, "I feel better working out at the health club every morning. I've got more energy, and my cholesterol's down. I have more to give to my kids and myself."

If you suspect that your partner is trying to undermine you—for example, even though he's well aware of your program, he stocks the refrigerator with chunky chocolate ice cream and brings home Krispy Kremes—here are specific ways to help him work through his feelings, bolster his confidence, and stay supportive. Most of these techniques are also adaptable for other saboteurs in your life:

Draft him. Ask him to coach you, and offer specific ideas about how he can help you, such as walking with you after dinner or before going to work in the morning. Perhaps he can take a swing dance class or join a bike club with you. Tell him how much you need his help to be successful.

Reassure him. Remind him how important he is to you and that your goal is a healthier, more vital you—not a replacement for him. Tell him about the energy the "new you" will bring to your relationship.

Communicate. When one wife put on substantial weight, she made comments such as "I really need to get back in shape." He'd respond, "Maybe you should," which she heard as criticism. She recalls, "I didn't have the smarts to say, 'I need your empathy. I want you to say, 'It must really be tough to get your body back after having babies, and when your hormones are out of kilter.' "

Renegotiate. Some couples have a silent understanding, such as, "If you don't bug me about my drinking, I won't bug you about your overeating." Or, "If you don't complain about me working on the computer or traveling all the time, I'll pretend I don't see you pigging out in front of the TV." When this goes on you're enabling each other, which isn't healthy for either of you or your relationship. He shouldn't be drinking so much and you shouldn't be eating so much. It's time to openly communicate and renegotiate these unspoken agreements. It's a wonderful opportunity for the relationship to grow.

Buddy up. Gently encourage him to change his eating and exercise habits too. Enlist his help in searching for healthy recipes, then create romantic dinners filled with good food and conversation. You can also entreat him to take a hike at your favorite park.

CHALLENGE YOUR OWN SELF TALK

At forty-six, an old friend of mine from college is a very successful Los Angeles executive recruiter—and a gorgeous woman. Divorced five years ago and very independent, she has always enjoyed a great deal of male attention. But she began to feel that she was not attracting men the way she used to.

"It hit me this summer," she told me. "At first I thought, 'It's just that people are vacationing, and there aren't as many men around.' But I'm realizing that the problem is I'm no longer as sexy. I know what men want, and my breasts aren't as high and full as they used to be, and my waist is thick."

I had a different view. I felt that the cultural message that sex appeal equals youth was so powerful that even this beautiful, smart, successful woman had bought it. She was putting herself down, and I told her so. Her bad feelings about herself had changed her demeanor. It had dampened her glow—and that was why fewer men were looking twice.

"I think that your assessment of yourself as less desirable affects your way of being," I said. "You dress differently than you normally do. You suddenly wear very plain clothes that play down your figure. They don't express who you are. I think that's sending a negative message to men."

She disagreed, arguing, "I know what men want and I used to have more of it."

"Since when have you defined yourself so much by what men want?" I asked her. "I think this attitude is holding you down. What would it be like to own what you're really about? You're a beautiful, smart, spunky, compassionate, achieving woman—and that was the way you came across until recently."

Part of sexual attraction is mystery, and that's what was missing in her. She had given up her more authentic way of being to please men, when it was that very authenticity, born of maturity, that had made her more exciting to them. As her true self, she was a more unpredictable presence. When we sacrifice our authenticity, it doesn't just stunt us, it stunts the men we're with. When we grow, it helps them grow. It can be scary to break out of the cage to become someone quite unexpected. Yet it's also wonderful— and it intrigues and challenges men.

How do you get back in touch with your authentic self? Use the following strategies for change to recognize how distorted thinking affects your behavior and the way others respond to you.

RECOGNIZE DISTORTION

Feeling less valuable as a woman, my friend exaggerated her flaws and ignored her considerable strengths. When you do that, you're less likely to feel that your body is worthy of tender loving care and act accordingly. To illustrate how off-base our own perceptions can be, I often ask women in my workshops to try the following exercise, which was developed by psychologist Roberta Sherman, Ph.D.

The task is to estimate the size of your waist—and then compare it with its actual size. To begin, take a ball of string and two paper clips. Judge the size of your waist by marking off how much string you think you'll need to circle it. Mark the spot on the string with one paper clip. Then wrap the string around your waist and mark its real size with the second paper clip.

Is your guess anywhere near the actual measurement? Most women find they grossly overestimate. Body distortion is an especially common form of negative body image that we all experience at times. For instance, when I tried this exercise myself, I calculated my own waist to be three inches larger than it really was.

Repeat this exercise on your hips, thighs, bust, and other parts of your body. Most people find there's a discrepancy between where they put the first paper clip and their true size.

One woman reported, "I estimated my waist and hips to be larger than they are. In contrast, I estimated my breasts to be smaller because I'm small chested to begin with. Since the ideal woman has a larger chest than I do, along with a smaller waist and hips, I'm not surprised at my estimate. I have a negative body image."

Someone else overestimated her measurements in order to avoid feeling disappointed. "I would rather think I'm fatter than I really am than imagine that I'm thinner than I am."

Another participant discovered that she didn't know her body as well as she thought. "My guesses ranged from overestimation to under. It was difficult for me to figure out the size by looking at the string. I'm definitely least comfortable with my hips. That goes back to my early years with Mom always seeming to focus on them. I'm concerned that my small waist makes my hips look so much bigger. I don't know how to dress to hide them. But it turns out that they really aren't that big. They are actually proportionate to the rest of my body. It was interesting to stand in front of the mirror this morning, trying to look at myself the way others do. I'm starting to work on seeing that I do look good and telling myself that all the time."

Someone who has small hips and accepts them noted, "I have an image of my waist that is bigger than it is. I think this exercise shows which parts of my body I truly accept and those I am usually pinching."

Chances are you're going to be surprised at how off-base many of your self-estimates are. Increasing awareness of your own distortions is an early step toward feeling better about yourself.

There is another distortion to watch out for, as well—the Swiss Cheese Phenomenon. A negative body image determines what experiences you notice and remember. If you believe you are not attractive, you are more likely to fixate on negative comments about your body than positive reactions to it, and attribute successes and failures in your life to your physical appearance, as in the statement "I didn't get the promotion because I'm less attractive than Amy."

Once a negative body image is formed, it is maintained even in the face of contradictory evidence. If you see yourself as fat and unappealing, you devalue compliments. You won't listen when your boyfriend tells you, "You look fabulous tonight." You'll say to yourself something like, "He's only saying that because he feels sorry for me." You feel uncomfortable hearing positive feedback from friends and others. It falls through the holes, like the holes in Swiss cheese. Negative feedback, however, no matter how much rarer and implausible, manages to stick. You also probably surround yourself with others who are obsessed with their appearance—and tolerate negative comments about how you look. Why? Because they confirm your own view.

STRATEGIES FOR CHANGE

If I told you to put on blue sunglasses, then placed a lemon in front of you and asked, "What color is it?" your answer would be, "It's greenish blue." When you have a negative body image, it's as if you're wearing blue sunglasses all the time. Your view of yourself is colored and skewed. The task is to challenge distorted thinking as well as faulty self-talk such as, "I can't go to the party. I'll die if anyone sees me at this weight." That kind of attitude not only affects your body image but also can lead to depression.

When you find yourself thinking this way, learn to have an inner dialogue with yourself, using the following techniques.

Visualize a Stop Sign and Tell Yourself to Stop

Identify negative thoughts about yourself that have become a bad habit. Then as they come up, halt them with your stop sign. Whenever you use your stop sign, be sure to replace the negative thought with a positive one.

Remind Yourself That You Are Wearing Sunglasses and May Not See Things Clearly

When younger men paid attention to her at swing dance sessions, Helen, fifty-three, had conversations with herself that ran something like: "How can I dance with him? I'm twenty years older than he is. Why would he even want to talk to me?" In fact, young men enjoy her. She's a good dance partner and is more interesting—and interested in listening to them—than women their own age. She says, "I've learned to tell myself to just shut up and have a good time." Which she does.

Challenge the Distortion

Do all others at the gym or pool look better than you do, or do they refuse to be deprived of activities on the grounds they are not perfect? If you tell yourself, "Only women with perfect bodies can work out in aerobics class," you must have a rare place in mind. Perfect 10s only exist in magazines. Ask yourself, "What is the evidence that my thinking is true?" and "What is the evidence that my thinking is not true?"

Think of What Has Worked in the Past

If you have a party coming up that you are dreading attending because of your weight, think of what you did at other parties to enjoy yourself. Perhaps you wore that knockout dress in your closet that makes you look so good. Or you focused on other guests at the party who always make you laugh.

Also reassure yourself. Say things such as, "It's hard to go to the party at this weight, but many other guests my age are struggling with their weight. I can get through this. I'm not going to die."

Learn a New Way to Talk About Your Body

When you speak of your body negatively, as in "My butt is so fat," you are talking negatively about yourself, and putting yourself down. Switch to affirmations instead, such as, "Weight training has really firmed up my arms."

Learn to Accept Compliments

Keep a journal in which you detail your responses to compliments. Recognize patterns in the way you react to good feedback—whether you tolerate cracks about how you look, rather than challenge them. You can pull out of the self-defeating cycle of poor body image, but you have to be deliberate about it.

Practice the art of being gracious and just say "thank you" when someone gives you a compliment, rather than devaluing the nice words. Don't add extras, such as, "Thank you, but my hair really doesn't look as good as it should." Or, "Yes, I now wear a size 10, but my stomach still hangs out." Or, "Yes, but I can't go to aerobics class until I lose another ten pounds." When you've accepted a compliment unequivocally, you've accepted a gift. There are good feelings for everyone—the recipient and the giver.

Get Out of the Cage and Do Something Different

My friend who believed that she'd lost her sex appeal has had a change of heart. What happened? She heard about an internet dating service that had great people, and she decided to try it. When she first got the idea, she complained that she never had to do that before.

"Well that's the way it is now," I told her. "The reality is people have time pressures, and the internet makes it easier and faster to find a date. And, at forty-six, maybe there aren't as many men out there."

Once she didn't see internet dating as a sign of failure anymore, she got moving. She has been dating like crazy ever since.

Will you spend the rest of your life making your body into a battleground, or will you take on the challenge of being deliberate about creating a lifestyle of self-care, where body acceptance can occur? Put yourself in situations where body acceptance, not a perfect body, is the important thing. Surround yourself with people who like and respect you no matter how you look.

7

ASSESS RELATIONSHIPS

*In giving up our impossible expectations, we become a lov-
ingly connected self, renouncing ideal visions of perfect
friendship, marriage, children, family life for the sweet imperfections of all-too-human relationships.*

—Judith Viorst,
Necessary Losses

Relationships form the context in which the midlife developmental
process occurs. Therefore, it is perfectly natural for them to change
at this time to reflect the shifts in you and your world. You may find
that you've outgrown certain roles, attitudes, and, in some cases,
even people. Real growth takes place when you can seize the opportunity to develop healthier, more satisfying relationships with
those you care about—relationships that encourage you to reach
your goals, feel good about yourself, and care for your body.

REWRITING THE MARRIAGE CONTRACT

Rebecca, forty-two, and her husband, Ed, forty-five, both MBAs,
met when he was in his last year at graduate school. They wed fifteen years ago after a whirlwind courtship.

"Here was this guy with a big smile, an open heart, and eyes filled with compassion. I took one look and said, 'Wow!' He had a joy and love for life that swept me away. I was so serious, and he was so much fun. He was all about relaxing and living fully every day. He showed me a side of men I'd never seen before. I came from a family where my dad was an angry alcoholic," explains Rebecca.

They settled in Atlanta, Ed's hometown, where life was a ball and he was Rebecca's golden boy. Ed's contacts, people skills, and business acumen led him to quick success as a venture capitalist. Rebecca, originally from Wisconsin, joined a consulting firm after completing her own graduate business degree. "We were incredibly sexual, and we were really good at having a great time. It was all parties and fun and games with Ed's circle of friends and business contacts. There was never a dull moment. The excitement was new to me, but I loved it," says Rebecca.

Five years later, after their first son arrived, however, life changed. Rebecca, determined to be a great mother, dropped her career to stay home full-time. Her role model was her own mom, who reared six children alone after Rebecca's father died when she was thirteen. "She gave up her life for us. I always called her the original Martha Stewart," says Rebecca, the youngest of the brood, who had the same exalted expectations for herself. "The reality of parenting hit me hard. I felt the focus of our life had to be the family now," she says. "The high life with Ed stopped being fun."

As Ed's company grew, Rebecca was his cheerleader. He continued to party for business and often took hunting and fishing trips with his friends. He worked so hard that Rebecca didn't object at first. But she gradually began to resent Ed's time away from home. "I probably let him think that he could do anything he wanted and I'd support it," muses Rebecca. "I did support it. He was romantic and fun. I had nothing to complain about. But I started to think, 'No, this is different. We have a family now.'"

Rebecca held her tongue, however, and her anger simmered.

She didn't know how a couple communicated, since she never saw it in her own parents. "I didn't know how to ask for what I wanted in a healthy way," she recalls. The more she poured herself into home and child, the more he focused on work. "We knew something was different, but we didn't realize how dangerous it was. I remember thinking one day, 'Being a cheerleader is not getting me what I want. I'll just be tougher and demand it.'"

She finally told Ed, "I've had it. You're away too much. You put your business first. I need you home at dinnertime. I need you to help care for our son." Instead of cooperation, she got anger and rebellion. Feeling attacked, Ed spent even less time at home. After their second son was born, Rebecca could feel them growing further and further apart. She became depressed. Ed, who had always been a social drinker, escaped through liquor.

Then Ed's mother and his best friend died within a few months of each other, and he experienced the possibility of failure for the first time when a business deal soured. Ed's drinking began to affect his work. "I think he didn't know how to say, 'I need you to support me, be close to me. Stop telling me that I'm a bad father. Help me,'" says Rebecca.

Not finding the support he needed at home, Ed had an affair. "I thought we invented love. I had no clue," Rebecca says. "He was such a romantic man and a decent person. We were best friends for so long. I knew him well enough to know it wasn't about sex. I think he wanted someone to tell him he was an okay guy. At home all I did was criticize."

Devastated at the betrayal, Rebecca's first thought was, "How did I get myself into this position? I left my career. I gave him a life where he could do anything he wanted, and he was seeing another woman. I willingly gave up a lot of my power to let him take control of our lives, and he did make it fun. But I didn't keep any leverage. It seemed okay at the time, but I think he lost respect for me. I was used to him taking the lead, but I gave up my voice in the process."

ED'S PERSPECTIVE

After graduate school Ed and Rebecca came back to his hometown, where he had all his friends. He made all the plans and told her, "Here's what we're doing. You've got to like this couple." He felt that if she loved him enough, she'd follow and do what he wanted convincing himself that every decision he made was for the good of their relationship and family. "I didn't plan things in partnership with Rebecca. Our marriage was a dictatorship, and I was the dictator" said Ed. He loved the outdoors, so instead of doing something that she might enjoy, such as going to a museum or out for a fancy dinner on weekends, he'd say, "We'll go camping." He thought he had the perfect wife, and Rebecca loved the life, although she lost some of her own personality. It got worse after the kids came along. Ed planned activities that Rebecca wouldn't attend.

"She was my best friend, but as the years went by, we started to lose our closeness because we didn't communicate. When I'd say, 'I'm going hunting this weekend,' she used to tell me, 'Go ahead and have a good time.' Before the children, she'd even come along. But then she started blowing up at me. She'd say, 'You're leaving us here.' "

And Ed would ask, "What happened to the person I married?"

When he came home from work, he wanted to hear "Did you have a tough day?"

The response he got was "Why are you two hours late?" He felt it was an attack on what he spent his whole life doing, which was working hard for their family. So he'd shoot back, "It's none of your business. I was making money for you." Or he'd retort, "What did you do today? The house is still a mess." Or, he'd work late again the next night.

He'd even make Rebecca feel that she was selfish to insist that he give up a fishing trip to be with the family. His attitude was, "Hey, I need this free time to get away from work." He observes, "If you want to face reality and talk about planning your life and your kids' future, you don't do that. I was really getting away from the responsibility of raising a family and being in a relationship with my best friend."

He started acting more and more selfishly. He wasn't going to be told that he wasn't a good man just because he drank beer and went out with the boys. At first he'd claim that social functions were part of business. He'd justify it by saying, "These guys go out and their wives don't yell at them."

Alcohol took it to the next level. When he was drinking he felt, "She's changed, I'll never do anything right. So I'll just go out and party. The kids are fine. They won't be affected just because our relationship isn't good."

Eventually, he met a younger woman. He felt she liked him for himself. If he didn't call for a few weeks, she didn't complain. She was ready to do anything he desired. "You start thinking that she's a good person to fulfill your plan with because she's different. But she's different because she doesn't come with the same responsibilities as your wife, who is the mother of your children and emotionally invested," he says.

So he fooled around. Inside he knew he was letting his family and himself down. Anytime those thoughts came into his head, it was time for a beer. He'd call his friends. Instead of drinking at 4 P.M., it became noon sometimes. He'd even call the woman he was seeing to come and join him with his friends. "I wasn't secretive—I was reckless. Instead of going to a business meeting, I'd go to a bar with her. I'd say to myself, 'I've got people who will cover for me.' I ran from family responsibility, a true relationship, my work, and before I knew it, the only person I was responsible for was the one who told me how nice I was. I went on for two years with this total self-absorption," Ed recalls.

"My father left my mother and married his secretary so that he could come home at night, find dinner waiting, and get sympathy from her. He wouldn't have to talk about the children or get yelled at. I was following directly in his footsteps."

Ed moved out. Rebecca blamed herself at first with, "It's me. This happened because I'm not as young and skinny as I used to be." She had gained thirty-five pounds since their marriage. As her anger at Ed increased, her rage consumed her. Following a lifelong pattern in response to stress, she'd have a drink or two, push food in her mouth, and not exercise.

Like many couples, Rebecca and Ed had a kind of unwritten agreement when they married. He expected her to be the doting wife who would raise the children, make a beautiful home, and allow him to be the fun guy. She expected him to be the good provider and a dad connected with the kids, who would put family first. "I wanted him to be everything my father wasn't. He wanted me to be what his mother wasn't," says Rebecca.

Such contracts can be beneficial if both people do their job and both are happy. Problems arise only when the deal doesn't work anymore—and when one person, usually the woman, is afraid to speak up. When Rebecca and Ed's high expectations of each other fell short and neither had the skills to deal with it constructively, their relationship fell apart. They needed to renegotiate their contract, but they didn't know how.

I find that many women lose themselves over the years, as Rebecca did. Believing that the only way they can stay in a relationship is to please the other person, they become what the spouse or partner wants them to be. Or they read what they think the other person wants and behave accordingly. It's a no-win situation, where the internal dialogue runs something like, "If I'm myself, I won't be able to keep this connection. But if I sacrifice my own needs to do what I think I have to in order to be a good wife or partner, I feel unhappy." In her book *Silencing the Self,* Dana Crowley Jack makes the case that women are more prone to depression than men are because they often hide their true selves in relationships.

During their separation, Ed agreed to go for counseling with Rebecca. Gradually, she began to recover her lost self. She began to reconnect with her girlfriends. She started to eat healthy and work out.

Ed turned around when his business hit rock bottom. At that time he realized that he had let down Rebecca and the kids just as his father had failed his family. "I didn't want to be like him, but I was doing exactly what he did, except I was spiraling down to alcoholism. It was a battle. I prayed for help, and the answer just came to me. It was, 'You need to drop everything, go to the person you love, and reprioritize your life before you become a statistic.'

"I think God said to me, 'If you want to keep going down that road, that's your choice, but you're failing.' It brought back to me how I felt when my father was never there for my ball games, and my mother didn't have a husband. We think as men that providing new cars and a big house is enough. If our wives are unhappy about that, we think we married the wrong wife because we can find women glad to hang out at bars with us and just have us bring home money. Finally, one night I drove to Rebecca's and told her, 'I know my life is out of control. I know alcohol is a large part of why. I'm ready to recommit to you.' "

They attended relationship classes—and still do. Ed, who went to AA briefly, participates in a support group of Christian men. He gave up drinking a year ago. He realized that if the relationship was to work, he had to come clean, do his share, and pray that Rebecca would forgive him.

"It will take her years to get back the trust she had. Understanding that has helped me be more honest myself," he says. "I've realized that I'm looking for forgiveness from God, and that forgiveness from her will come. Our relationship can be better than it was before.

"What you really want is your friend who holds you at the end of a tough day. The only way to get that back is to communicate and know each other. Men don't want to say to their wives, 'I know you're mad, but here's why I'm late,' because they almost feel it's weak. So instead of stopping it right there, they storm out. Communication is sharing things with your partner, and men have a tough time understanding that."

Rebecca returned to her faith, which became a lifeline for her. "Whatever your spirituality, you need a foundation," she observes. She and Ed joined a church community with many people their own age who weren't shy about sharing their problems. They feel accepted there. They have also renegotiated what the term *commitment* means. "Are you committed to your job—or to your kids? We decided we had to be committed to each other first and foremost. We were two injured people who decided to rebuild together," says Rebecca.

And their expectations are rooted in reality, which gives them new respect for each other. Rebecca sees now that Ed is a human being, not a god. "I wanted security. I expected him to meet all my needs and make my life great, but no one person can fulfill all my needs. I've found other places to meet my needs, such as church and friends. I can also go work out. I'm learning how to soothe myself and take care of myself." She's also looking for part-time work that will allow her to use her considerable skills.

Her strength awes Ed. "It was incredible to him that I survived all this and still truly loved him," she says.

Do you have an unspoken marriage contract that needs to be revisited? Sometimes the agreement is a variation of Rebecca and Ed's, or it takes other forms. I've seen situations where the woman wants to get out in the world more, as her career or interests rev up in midlife. At the same time, his career is winding down, and he's tired of traveling or spending so much time on business. They're out of sync and need to rewrite their agreement.

Change can lead to growth, and one of the neat things about growth is that it forces you to develop new skills. You may become responsible for fewer household chores and invest more time in developing your business skills. Your husband may develop more skills of leisure, learning to cook and to nurture. The important thing to remember is that both of you can flourish in satisfying new roles.

REVITALIZING A TIRED MARRIAGE

In other midlife marriages, the problem isn't the contract but boredom with the relationship. I think that many affairs occur because someone else out there looks more interesting than your spouse. But often the person you're with is very interesting. You're just both stuck in a routine. To explore the possibilities, you need to get out of the cage together, follow interests and passions, and do things you wouldn't normally do. Becoming adventurous together stirs excitement in a marriage.

For example, one wife in her late forties became interested in the work of young, emerging contemporary artists. She began to visit museums and galleries to learn more about them, coming home to tell her husband, a tax consultant, about what she saw. Soon he became intrigued, as well. They started collecting art. "We were a great team," she explains. "I did the research and scouted out artists I thought were great. He wasn't interested in art history, but he had a fabulous eye for what was a good painting or drawing. He'd pick out their best work and negotiate the price with the gallery. He also had the guts to buy when I'd get cold feet and obsess, 'How can we spend money on this. My mother will think we're crazy.' We had such fun for years and years."

Although she did not develop this interest specifically to spice up her marriage, their joint effort in fact opened up a whole new world for them in midlife. There were always exhibitions they wanted to see, even on vacation trips. They subscribed to an auction catalog, an art magazine, and read the arts section of the newspaper with new eyes. When articles mentioned an artist whose work hung on their wall, they felt thrilled.

There are many ways to discover new dimensions of your relationship as empty nest approaches, or if it is already here. Take a course together, volunteer together, go ballroom dancing together, get active in a political campaign and/or your place of worship, or take bridge lessons. You can even pursue interests separately, then come together to share information and enthusiasm and learn from each other. When you are both growing, the two of you have a lot more to talk about than taxes and the kids.

ENERGIZING YOUR SEXUAL RELATIONSHIP

Your sex life can also get tired in midlife, yet this is a time when your sexual relationship can grow and move in healthy new directions.

The great thing about midlife is it's a chance to reach deeper levels of connection and satisfaction. "The best sexual connections actually happen at this time when midlife partners (and even older couples) have learned how to welcome soulful sexual energy into their lives," says Lana Holstein, M.D., author of *How to Have Magnificent Sex*. She has found that women often worry less about how they look and men worry less about how they're doing. Then they can ask instead, "How am I connecting? How well can I love this man in my life and allow him to see the inner me?" Letting someone see inside you, as well as looking inside him, takes the sexual experience to another level.

So often when a couple make love they are out of sync. One person is worrying about the to-do list and the other's mind is at the office. Something as simple yet profound as soul gazing, a technique that Holstein and her husband David teach in their sexuality courses, brings you both into the moment. It helps you focus in just two or three minutes. Says Holstein, "It's so valuable to have a method to create the emotional container for the two of you before beginning to touch each other's bodies and stimulate each other sexually. It's also very intimate to look into your partner's eyes as you're making love and feel awed by how special it is to bring him into your body. That really adds to your sexual connection. This is lovemaking at a level of maturity that I think couples can reach as they live together and make love together over time."

Soul gazing is very powerful and actually comes from an ancient view of sexuality called Tantra. You can try it yourself. Sit across from each other at the beginning of a sexual encounter, hold hands with your left hand up to represent receiving, and your right hand down on your partner's hand to represent giving. Then look into each other's eyes and breathe together. Don't talk, because if you do, you're likely to talk about money and the kids.

After going through so much together, the ups and downs of raising children, and grieving losses, you can feel a deep level of closeness that you never had before. This can be expressed through your body during sex. The intimacy and trust that you've built can lead to more creative lovemaking, taking more risks, and opening your body and self up to your lover. This communication of acceptance and love of each other's aging bodies can lead to a more positive body image for both of you.

THE CONFIDENCE FACTOR

As you mature, there is also a confidence that seeps into your sense of self. And when you feel deserving of a pleasurable sexual experience, and know who you are and what you want, you can ask for it. Informing your partner of what works for you is crucial. You're not going to get to exceptional sex by making your partner guess what you want.

Many women were raised to be shy or worry that they'll wound a partner's ego if they make a suggestion. But there are ways to make suggestions without hurting your partner's feelings. Direct, specific feedback from you enables your partner to please you and leads to excitement about the capacity to bring you pleasure. Say "I loved it when you gently caressed my nipples." Or, "It excited me when you told me you loved me as you stimulated me." Such specific statements lead to more pleasure for your partner and more feelings of competency and effectiveness. Instead of hurting feelings, directness boosts your partner's ego. Men get really excited when they feel potent and able to bring you pleasure.

What if you have no partner? If you are interested in attracting one, don't avoid sex or sexual thoughts. Excluding sensuality and sexuality from your life turns off your feminine sexual essence. Instead, read novels that include sexual references and passages and books about sexuality.

I also encourage you to explore masturbation if you feel comfortable with it. Masturbation allows you to discover what type of stimulation pleases your body the most. If you don't want to masturbate, that's fine too, but read those sexy books and watch those sexy movies. You don't have to become celibate mentally, as well as physically, just because you don't have a partner now. Hopefully, someday soon you will have a partner again.

Express your sensuality through the way you move, the way you smell and touch those around you. Communicate what you want, whether it's the type of food you're in the mood for or what kind of foreplay you're fantasizing about. Let your joy and radiance come through. Don't be afraid to put on some sexy sandals, try a great new fragrance, buy a teddy, comment on your lover's cologne. If a man smells great, tell him. Sensuality is paying attention to your senses, appreciating what you look at, what you smell, what you hear. Get in the habit of saying, "I love your deep voice." Or, "Nobody smells like you." When your sensuality is alive, you're much more likely to get a response from men around you.

As for your midlife body, it's great if you're in shape, but it doesn't mean that you can't have good sex if you have big hips or are overweight. What counts is that midlife can be a time when you feel freer, which can affect your body image—and your sexual experience—in a very positive way.

"Most men are delighted as you get turned on sexually. They tell me, 'I am not looking at her cellulite when I make love. I'm attracted by how aroused she's becoming.' They'll also say, 'I don't look like I did when I was twenty or thirty either. I understand that, and I very much want to make love to this woman.' It's a matter of being able to move away from concentration on body details and begin to say, 'What I'm exposing is my soul.' And that is always deeper and more meaningful than a superficial connection," says Holstein.

When you enjoy each other outside the bedroom, you increase enjoyment inside the bedroom. Be deliberate about setting aside time to be alone together and relax. Make a date for frequent Saturday nights out and an occasional weeknight dinner without the kids. Suggest, "Next Wednesday night I'd really like you to go with me to the town meeting. We'll get a sitter, and afterward, let's get a motel room and be romantic." Pull out a sexy negligee and wear it. Says one husband, "Before the kids, my wife used to call me and say, 'I'll get off at 11:45 A.M. Let's have lunch today.' I want her to do that kind of thing again. Who cares if she doesn't have the body she used to. It's in the eyes of the beholder. My wife is the same woman I fell in love with."

Good sex is a birthright. It's part of having a vital sense of self. If your sexual interactions are not the way you want them, there are therapists, books, and other resources to help. In midlife, men may have sexual problems, such as erectile dysfunction, but there are better solutions than ever before, such as Viagra and testosterone replacement. There is also help for body changes in women that may interfere with sexual pleasure.

Energizing your sex life can be fun. To improve your tennis game, you take lessons, practice, and maybe work with a pro. When it comes to sex, however, it's common to think, "I already should know about this." Instead, think of sex as a skill to enhance, and practice, practice, practice.

DEVELOPING AN ADULT RELATIONSHIP WITH PARENTS

I once treated a forty-four-year-old computer industry executive named Lydia whose weight had gone up and down for years. One of the things that she and her best friend had in common was anger toward their parents. They both nursed their rage, trading stories of their grievances virtually every time they got together until the friend's father was diagnosed with terminal cancer.

As he lay dying, the friend began to spend a great deal of time with him. "I feel that I'm starting to forgive my father," she confided one night over dinner with Lydia. The latter felt so shocked and threatened that she proceeded to stuff herself for the rest of the night. She ate all the rolls in the basket and topped the meal off with banana cream pie. What was going on? Suddenly she had lost her partner in blaming, who had served an important purpose. As long as the two of them clung to blame, they didn't have to take action to deal with their problems. But the friend's ability to change and reconnect with her father put pressure on my patient to look at her relationship with her own parents.

A few days later, Lydia told me about the evening. As we talked, she began to realize that she and her friend had become stuck in the same way. The friend was finally letting her anger go and moving on. Lydia, however, refused to do that unless her own mother and father admitted how badly they had treated her.

To help her understand what she was doing to herself, I told her this Buddhist story:

> In medieval times, there was a knight who was shot with an arrow. Furious with pain, he vowed, I will not take this arrow out until I find out who shot it at me. The knight wound up dying of an infection.

"My fear for you is that you're like the knight. You are going to die of an infection because your parents are not going to tell you what you want to hear. They did make mistakes and did harmful things. But you're now forty-six years old and they're in their late seventies. They're trying to reconnect with you and have invited you for Easter dinner," I said.

"I just can't go. I don't like being around them," she insisted.

"How long is their penance?" I asked. "There's a point where not only are they paying a price, but you are too."

Lydia's price was a hostile attitude that turned people off and an inability to sustain relationships with men. To fill the void, she turned to food instead of people. Part of our work together involved increasing the time she spent with others, and getting her to start dating. But she wasn't going to be able to stop overeating and really let someone in emotionally until she dealt with her rage toward her parents—especially her father, who had criticized her unmercifully as a child and made her feel unaccepted. Having experienced so much of it, she unconsciously felt comfortable with criticism. She chose critical men, then said, "See, they are all alike." When she met someone who sincerely liked her just as she was, she'd manipulate and set him up with statements like, "Did you notice that I'm always late?" Then if he replied, "You know what, you are late," she'd insist, "Men are always critical. Relationships never work." In fact, she made sure they didn't work.

Unfortunately, Lydia's stubbornness won out. She refused to work on her problems with her parents. Although she saw how healing forgiveness had been for her friend, she didn't feel ready to pull out that arrow.

Many people grow up and do develop healthier relationships with their parents in midlife. They let go of their anger, accepting that nobody's perfect. Often they've raised their own children and realize the mistakes they've made themselves, which helps them to forgive. They can give up complaints such as, "My mother neglected me because she hated me," because they can now realize, "My mother had a hysterectomy during that period. She did kind of abandon me, but it wasn't because she hated me. It was because she was depressed."

A child has an egocentric view, thinking, "It's always about me. Mom and Dad divorced because of me." An adult realizes that they divorced because they didn't get along and couldn't work out their problems.

Are you able to stand back and look at how incredibly complicated relationships, as well as the motives behind behavior, are for people? A childish view is, "Mom was always critical of my body because she thought I was unattractive." An adult reaction is, "I've learned more about my mother. She was an overweight kid who felt a lot of shame about her body. She wanted to make sure it didn't happen to me, so she focused, probably too much, on my weight and shape. But the motive wasn't that she hated me. She loved me. Unfortunately what she did was not helpful."

Forgiving your parents doesn't mean you don't still have some negative feelings toward them. But often you're able to say, "This is who my mother is at seventy-nine. At her age, she may never change. But I may have to change the way I respond to her or I keep this arrow lodged in me. So I'm going to handle her differently. If she talks about weight I'll confront her or make a joke, and move on."

It's important to let go of childish ways of viewing parents and see them for who they are because hanging on to old business keeps you closed to healthy relationships with others and yourself. If your father left when you were six, hanging on to rage at how he abandoned you can fuel a compulsion to look for him in romantic relationships. Too often women choose men to re-create relationships with their parents. Unconsciously they feel comfortable with people who don't fulfill their needs.

You can't control how you grew up, but you can be courageous and surround yourself with different people now. Growing up means holding out for men who can teach, mentor, and encourage you—who are different from the nonnurturing types you usually choose. Dating men who don't nurture you is accepting what you always got—not much. To make up for it, you may overeat, drink, and/or spend a lot of money on things you don't need.

When you relate to your parents more like a grown-up, you can often move from being a little girl to being a woman in other ways as well. Are you still overeating to get back at your mother because she always wanted you to be thin and continually asks what size you are? That's not a healthy relationship. You might be geographically separate—you might live in Albuquerque and she's in Philadelphia—but you're not emotionally separate. You need to honor all the wisdom you have at this point in your life, begin to relate to your parents in a different way, and finally create your own vision for your body.

I've found that forgiving your parents can lead you to look and feel sexier. I see patients who start treatment wearing sweatpants that are way too big for them and oversized sweatshirts decorated with motifs like Winnie the Pooh. They overeat, don't exercise, have made their bodies round and asexual—and they're still mad at their mothers. They handle anger and present themselves in a childlike way, although they operate responsibly and do a great job in other areas, such as raising their kids or running a business. But they don't know how to deal with a demanding mother as one adult to another.

In such cases, a woman often says, "I don't feel sexy at all." Somewhere inside she feels like a child—and little girls aren't supposed to be sexy. If you can't set boundaries and speak up to Mom, chances are you can't say to your husband, "I want to be touched," and you can't initiate sex.

As we work together, I challenge these women to come up with new ways to handle anger at a parent. Suddenly they start making time to exercise and their bodies take on more definition. They dress differently, too, replacing oversized apparel with clothes such as sweater sets, which fit better and reveal their shape. As they become more fully formed women, their sexuality emerges.

Remember that your parents most likely did the best they could with the resources they had. Resentment and bitterness will get you nowhere. Forgive—and acknowledge the positives from your family. Then enjoy the freedom letting go of grudges brings.

GETTING PAST GRUDGES

I've developed this technique to help patients who are immobilized by grudges against parents or others. I suggest that they pick out a date a month or two away. If the date is June 1, I then say, "You can be angry at your mother because all she cares about is your weight until July first. Between now and then, you are going to either think about how angry she makes you or write about it every day for ten minutes. On July first, however, you're going to light a candle, imagine your anger within the flame, and blow it out. When you do, you're going to let that anger go for good. It's done. From that moment on, you cannot talk to me or anyone else about it. If you start to do that, you're going to tell yourself to stop—because talking about it feeds it and makes it grow."

I've found that telling someone to be mad has a paradoxical effect. The anger loses its appeal when the person is told to vent it. Patients often come in and tell me, "I've been doing this for twenty-two days and I'm so sick of writing about how furious I am at my parents." Or they realize the distortion in their view.

If you haven't been able to move beyond a grudge, try picking out a date yourself. This technique may work well for you. It is also effective for people who are plagued by guilt. If someone can't forgive herself for giving up a baby for adoption years ago, I'll say, "That's a big decision you made and you have many complicated feelings about it, but how long is your penance going to be? It's been twenty-two years." Often the exercise leads them to come back with reasons why the guilt needs to stop. They might say, "I did this, but at the time I had no choice. Since then I've had two children. I've been a good mother."

TAKE INVENTORY OF FRIENDSHIPS

When Ed moved out during their separation, Rebecca realized for the first time that she really had no friends to confide in and trust. Her social circle consisted mainly of Ed's friends and their wives. Would they keep her secrets? She also wanted them to continue to love Ed, and she felt guilty complaining about him to them. She couldn't turn to her family because she felt she had let them down. Most of her siblings were divorced, and she was considered the family success story. Her elderly mother's hopes and dreams had centered on her.

Frightened, lonely, and seeking to educate herself about alcoholism and infidelity, she turned to the internet to do research. In the process, she stumbled onto a chat room, which led to an email friendship with another wife whose high-profile husband was an alcoholic. "I had no one to talk to but her. I called her my angel, my invisible friend. I was a zombie, barely able to communicate, but she was patient and listened," recalls Rebecca.

Eventually, Rebecca realized that she needed more. Her husband was out of control, and she had to be the anchor for her family. She felt that she had to prove to her kids and herself that she could be in charge, and that meant gathering allies. For the first time she reached out to a friend and broke down. "I told her, 'My marriage is probably over, and I need someone to help me.' Luckily I picked a wonderful person to be my support. She took care of me, let my kids stay over, and listened to me. She was there when I needed her," recalls Rebecca.

When I see women in their forties and fifties who are struggling in midlife, isolation is sometimes part of the problem, especially if they're suffering from depression. They may be shamed by a marital breakup or they're embarrassed about how empty and lost they feel because their kids have left home. But they don't share it with friends or their spouses. They just drink a little more or sleep a lot or think, "All of a sudden I've got all these wrinkles and put on weight," which leads them to cut back socially.

Yet interaction with other people is exactly what they need. As you tell your story to a friend, a new story forms. When you confess, "I feel unattractive and old and matronly," a friend is likely to assure you, "I know just what you mean. I felt that way three weeks ago." And as you talk the experience through, you move into a new space. She might propose, "Why don't we try to do something about this together? The Diabetes Marathon is in April. Why don't we start training for it?" Before you know it, that sadness you felt starts to dissipate and you reclaim your energy by moving on.

Do you have a friend in whom you can safely confide and who lives near enough to be available regularly? Now is a time to take stock of your friendships and ask, "Do I have friends who meet my needs?"

In middle age, many women realize how out of touch they are with serious parts of themselves, such as how they really feel about their social lives. As they get older, they're pickier about who they spend time with. They realize that they won't be here forever. A theme that has emerged in midlife groups is that age has a way of pushing you to reconnect with who you really are, your core self, that person you were before you worked or had family obligations, which leads you to reevaluate what you want in a friend. For instance, several of my workshop participants have mentioned that associating with important people is less appealing now. One woman explained, "When I was younger I would join a committee to work for the symphony because I knew a particular woman was on it and I wanted to get into her group of friends. I have no interest in that now. I no longer choose friends based on prestige or money. I want to be with good people who love and accept me."

Someone else commented, "I'm more into quality, not quantity, now. When I was in my twenties and thirties, I wanted a million friends. I wanted to be friends with all my kids' friends' parents. I wanted everyone to like and approve of me. Now I just want a few very close friends."

Do these comments resonate for you? Slow down and think about it. How much time do you spend with people you really want to be with? Says a teacher and mother of three, "At forty-four, I want to be a good mother. I also want to be good at my work, and there's not a lot of time for much else. I ask myself, 'How often do I see people out of habit and convenience and because I want to be liked or because I'm afraid of hurting others' feelings?' "

Honor the fact that you have limited time, and prioritize the people you want to spend it with. Make a list of people you'd like to see more of. Call one of them today. Get creative about squeezing in face-to-face time. For example, you might schedule your manicures together, or walk together on Saturdays, combining talk with exercise.

Has your confidante moved away, or do you need more friends who are life-affirming and supportive? Then keep your eye out for new people who can fill in such gaps. How about friendships with men? They offer a different perspective, and it's enriching to have male friends you can talk to and feel validated by. As for women friends, don't limit yourself to those your own age. Older friends offer wisdom and the benefit of experience, while younger friends bring fresh ideas and can lead you to new activities and possibilities. One woman, fifty, a dedicated volunteer and full-time mother of three, had the time of her life on a cross-country skiing trip with four women ten to fifteen years younger. "I felt so flattered when they invited me, and I loved it," she reported. "I'd never have done it without them. I trained for weeks to get myself in shape, worrying that I couldn't keep up with them. But I did fine. I was sore afterward, but I know how to train better now. I can't wait for next time."

Get in touch with a couple of friends you'd like to see more of, especially those who share new interests that you and your partner are developing. They can enrich your marriage. If you can't think of any, be on the lookout.

MATURING AS A FRIEND

A woman in one of my groups observed, "It's not always easy being in relationships with people, but I think loving others is the most important thing you can do. People are human, so they sometimes get on your nerves or disappoint you, but they also come through for you when you make a mistake, your husband leaves, or you didn't get the promotion you expected.

"As I get older I'm easier on my friends. I don't expect so much affection or attention. As I'm that way with them, I notice that I'm getting easier on myself."

When you reach your forties and fifties, you realize that there are no perfect people. With that in mind, I think we need to let go of childish ways of dealing with each other and handle mistreatment by friends like adults. Part of growing up is accepting that we're big girls and can take care of ourselves. People are human, and unfairness will happen. We have to develop skills so that even when someone is being unkind to us we can communicate, and go home to deal with the incident without raiding the freezer.

This story, told by Leslie, a workshop participant, is a perfect example. After eating in a seafood restaurant, Leslie got sick from the food. Since she had liked the place in the past, she gave it a second chance. But she became ill again. Sometime later, a former coworker proposed that they have dinner together at the same restaurant. Leslie explained, "I used to love their menu, but I don't want to go there anymore. Getting sick twice is my quota."

The friend retorted, "Listen, I want to go there. It's not always about you."

Shocked by the hostility, Leslie got so upset that she went home and ate a box of donuts.

As soon as Leslie concluded the story, someone else in the workshop chimed in sympathetically, "That friend sounds like a bitch." Others murmured their agreement.

But I responded, "Wait a minute. Let's take a look at this."

We're not little kids. We're grown women. We need to learn to handle others' mistreatment or anger without using it as an excuse to overeat. We can't call up all our pals and have five people bad-mouth this person. We have to be able to contain the incident and cope with it rather than blame someone else's nastiness for our bingeing, excessive drinking, or perpetual unhappiness.

The restaurant story illustrates when it's time to sit down with a friend and talk about the relationship. It may not be right away. You may have to say, "Let's wait until we calm down. We need a little more space from each other. Let's have coffee next week to talk things out."

There's a real opportunity for growth in such cases. Usually people don't make such a strong statement based on one incident. When you do sit down and talk, you may discover that you have been too self-centered in this relationship. Or you're not self-centered and it's the first time you've spoken up for yourself. If you automatically react by telling your friends how awful this person is (and they agree) and you never directly deal with the person, a chance to learn and grow has been lost.

LEARN HOW TO GET WHAT YOU WANT

Think about a troubling situation in your life that forces you to deal with a person you care about. Whether it involves a spouse, boyfriend, family member, or friend, do you know how to get what you want effectively? Misguided beliefs and/or lack of key relationship skills sometimes stop us from getting our needs met. Following are two ways to change that.

SET BOUNDARIES

A boundary is a limit that defines you and separates you from others. It helps shape relationships so that your desires are recognized and respected. Like Rebecca, however, women often don't know how to set limits or wait too long to do so.

"I wish she had forced the issue quicker, instead of taking a backseat and saying, 'He'll come out of this. He'll realize that running around with his buddies isn't right,' " says Ed.

Ed was basically a good guy who knew the importance of responsibility, but Rebecca didn't know him well enough to realize that he'd rebel against being told what to do. She needed to sit down with him early and ask, "How can we work it out together so that we have enough family time?" Only then could they negotiate.

Sometimes boundaries have to change because life throws a curve. An administrator in one of my workshops had an unspoken contract with her husband that said she would not only care for the kids but also help out his parents. And it was okay with her until she developed severe arthritis. Although she was a very giving person, she had to stop supervising her in-laws' medical and other needs because she had to take care of herself.

"I've been caring for other people my whole life, but I can't do it to the degree I did before," she explained. "Now I have a chronic illness that I have to deal with." Yet she feared her husband's reaction if she told him she was quitting her job as caretaker.

The first step she needed to take was to acknowledge that they had both silently agreed to this arrangement. She then needed to tell her husband, "And now I can't do it anymore because I'm sick. How can we work it out so that your mother gets good care?"

After she and her husband discussed the situation, they decided to make the medical appointments in the late afternoon and evening. Although she would do the scheduling, her husband and their teenaged daughter could then take the elderly couple to the doctor's office.

Boundary issues can also arise when a husband starts a business and suddenly works at home. If you have a home office yourself or if you're a full-time homemaker, it may drive you crazy when he walks in to chat, as if he's going to the office watercooler, or he wants to have lunch with you every day in the kitchen.

How do you handle the intrusion on your turf? Instead of overeating and gaining ten pounds, set limits and figure out a schedule. You might say, 'From eight to twelve I need my space. I want to be alone to go about my work, phone calls, my stuff, my life." It doesn't matter what you do during your time; even if you're watching soap operas, having him around can feel like an intrusion. Maybe you can then negotiate having lunch together once or twice a week.

Often the same issue comes up when men retire. Some want their wives to become their mothers, to walk with them and cook their breakfast. There's a period of transition, and the dialogue is the same: "We have to set up a schedule."

We also need to set boundaries with others in the course of daily life. A friend of mine, a divorced mother of two in Connecticut, sets boundaries exceptionally well. Aware that she was attending a wedding in Boston on the same weekend that a Boston fund-raiser I helped organize was taking place, I asked her to buy a ticket and attend. Since it was for an important professional cause, she said, "Sure." Then she discovered that the relative she was staying with that weekend actually lived ninety minutes away from the city. She'd have to travel three hours round trip. She left this message on my answering machine: "Ann, I'll buy a ticket, but I won't be there. I wanted to attend to give you moral support, but the long commute would make the weekend crazy for me."

Many women in the same situation would feel, "No matter what, I have to do it." I sometimes feel that way myself. But my friend has good boundaries, a real definition of what's acceptable and not acceptable for herself with men, with her kids, with everyone. She takes care of herself, and it shows. I told her, "This is one of the reasons you're a role model for me."

SEND A STRONG SIGNAL

Sometimes what blocks people from getting what they want is the expectation that others should know what they need without being told. We all wish others could just read our minds and know how to support us. But the reality is we have teach them, which is why you need to ask yourself, "Have I sent a strong enough signal? Does this person know what I want and expect?"

Pam, forty-one, almost wrecked her relationship with her in-laws by expecting them to be mind readers. Pam, who is Jewish, and her husband, who is not, agreed to celebrate both of their holidays but to bring up the children in her religion. Her husband's parents respected and accepted their decision. Pam's son's bar mitzvah was scheduled to take place in Chicago. Her father died several months before, and she was particularly anxious for her in-laws to be there. She wanted her son to have a grandfather present.

Her in-laws, who are in their seventies and live in Arizona, faced a conflict. Another grandchild, who lives in New York, was graduating from high school on the Sunday of the same weekend. Their solution was to attend the Saturday morning bar mitzvah ceremony, then fly to New York later that afternoon. They would skip the Saturday night bar mitzvah party. Their compromise devastated Pam. She said, "I wish you'd stay for the party and leave for the graduation on Sunday morning."

They replied, "We wish we could too, but we have to go."

Pam could have spoken more clearly and explained, "This is the first major event without my father, and my son and I need your support. I realize that it isn't easy to attend all these events in one weekend. But I really need you to stay Saturday night and come to the party so that my son will have a grandfather there. You can always take the flight in the morning. It would mean a lot to me."

But Pam refused to do that. When I asked why, she answered,

"They should have known." But they didn't. You have to teach people how to support you. When you do, the chances increase that you'll get what you need.

I told her, "Spell it out. Tell them, 'This is really important. I need you to do this. I'll be glad to get all the information on Sunday morning flights for you so that you won't miss the graduation.' "

After thinking it over, Pam decided to take my advice, and her in-laws agreed to change their plans. She got what she wanted.

We can also make incorrect assumptions about people that may lead to misunderstandings. Pam felt hurt that her in-laws didn't fly in for her father's funeral, sending flowers instead. Later, when she visited them for Christmas, they never mentioned her father's death. Pam saw it as an example of their coldness, as compared to her own warm family. I suggested that she tell her in-laws, "I felt hurt that my father's death was never mentioned. I'm the type of person who really needs your support when a loss occurs. I need to talk about it because that helps me."

Sometime later, I received an email from Pam that said, "I talked to my in-laws. They told me that three of their friends had died since summer. They felt overwhelmed when my father also died. They knew how upset I was, and thought that I might need a break at Christmas to just have some fun. That's why they never mentioned my father. But they were thinking of me and they prayed for him."

Pam discovered that her in-laws were actually far more caring than she realized. We can remain small-minded and say, "If people loved me, they'd read my mind and see that I'm upset." But in real relationships we have to speak up. That increases the chances that we'll get the support we need.

THE BOTTOM LINE

Is there anything more important in your life than your relationships with loved ones and friends? Do some of those relationships need to change to give voice to the person you are and allow you to move ahead? It's frightening to venture out of the cage, take risks, explore new limits and terrain. It's easier to leave relationships alone rather than set new boundaries or get closer to others.

After I finished lecturing in Australia last year, I spent a day hiking in the Raintree Forest with a sixty-five-year-old Aboriginal guide named Daisy. We would hike for a few hours, then Daisy and I would stop, and she would teach me about the Aboriginal culture. During one of the stops, Daisy shared that the Aboriginal people were a hunting and gathering society. She turned to me and said, "What are you hunting for at this point in your life, Ann, and who are you gathering around you?"

It was a simple, yet profound question that I spent months thinking about. It may be time for you to ask yourself this question. What are you hunting for at this point in your life? Is it just the "perfect body," or are you yearning for meaning and more adventure? Who are you gathering around you—people who can enjoy and support your changing body and evolving self or those who seem overly invested in you staying the same? Change, even good change, causes anxiety and doesn't always feel good. Yet developing healthier relationships can help heal body image struggles. When you feel loved and supported, it's easier to accept your body.

8

LEARN FROM OTHER CULTURES

When one woman puts her experience into words, another woman who is kept silent, afraid of what others will think, can feel some validation. And when that second woman says aloud "yes—that was my experience too," the dream of common language is realized in that moment.

—Carol Christ,
Diving Deep and Surfacing

In a study that compared body image and self-image among African-American, Asian, and Caucasian girls, African-American girls were found to have the most positive body image. Their images were so much healthier than those of Asian and Caucasian girls that the researchers decided to talk to them and find out why. The researchers discovered that when African-American girls look out into the world, they find few women of their race who are considered ideal beauties. In response, they create their own ideal, based on their personal physical attributes.

The positive body image of African-American girls continues into adulthood. Virtually all of the research shows that adult African-American women have the best body image, as well. We need to pay attention to African-American women. Creating our own ideal of beauty is a protective factor against body dissatisfaction.

A three-day workshop I conducted for *O* magazine at Canyon Ranch in December 2001 explored what we can learn not only from African-American women but also from a range of diverse cultures and ethnic groups. The true wonder of the United States is that we are a melting pot unlike any other nation in the world. We—or our parents, grandparents, or great- (or great-great-) grandparents—came from someplace else, with the exception of Native Americans. The goal of the workshop was to explore the effect of our various heritages of origin—as well as the impact of our dominant American culture—on how we feel about our bodies. Participants, who ranged in age from the twenties to sixties, were Caucasian, African-American, Hispanic, and Asian. At the first meeting, I asked them to introduce themselves, talk about their backgrounds, and what it means to be a woman in their culture or heritage. A common thread that ran across ethnic and racial lines seemed to emerge rather quickly: a sense of discontinuity.

Years ago, women used to sit down together, sharing family history and stories of how to be female. These deeply authentic stories, which were handed down through the generations, provided a model of womanhood—which nourished identity, community, and security. Today, however, instead of being shaped by such stories, women often fill themselves up with stories from the outside. As a consequence, we lose rich meaning in our lives. In my own practice, I've found that teenagers I treat don't know much about their backgrounds or even their grandparents. They know more about their teen idols' families, and they take on their stories to develop an identity.

We also used to glance around and see what women looked like in our neighborhoods, and at school. Some women were considered more attractive than others, but they were real people with real bodies. It enriched us to know that we were like them, or would be when we grew up. But real role models have been replaced by airbrushed images from the media. Many of us have bought into them, fantasizing, "If I look like this woman on TV or in this magazine, I'll be happy and successful." Because few of us can equal her, we feel bad about ourselves. As a Korean-American woman in her late twenties summed it up, "The negative feelings and ideas I have about my body are not simply because of my ethnic and cultural background. They come precisely from these dual pulls of being both Korean and American."

I suggested that we make sense of this theme of discontinuity, caused largely by globalization and mobility in the modern world, and pursue it as the theme of the workshop. I proposed, "Let's get rid of the television set and computer. Let's sit here and engage in the age-old ritual of storytelling. Let's share stories about what it means to be an African-American woman or a Hispanic woman, or someone of another background. Let's talk about the traditions we've been taught that play a role in how we see ourselves, compare these stories, and learn from them."

What followed was a fascinating journey of discovery. Here are highlights that emerged in the workshop—and in the voices of women in research I conducted on the same issues, at around the same time.*

DIFFERING IDEALS OF FEMALE BEAUTY

I found that each ethnic group represented in the workshop was taught a rich stereotype of the ideal woman in its culture. However, this model usually differed dramatically from the American ideal. The clash often caused confusion and fed the sense of disconnection.

---

*Women who are not identified as workshop participants answered an online survey through *O* magazine about the effects of ethnicity on body image.

HISPANIC

Although there are variations in Hispanic culture depending on the country of origin and other factors, Latina women in the workshop learned that curves, large breasts, big, round hips, and a small waist are desirable. They were taught to look sexy, have children (that's what the hips are for), nurture and take care of others, not work outside the home, and be submissive to men. In contrast, American culture tells them to look ultrathin, be independent, make their own money, and take charge of their sexuality.

A twenty-five-year-old Ecuadorian-Mexican woman in the workshop, who moved to New York with her mother when she was twelve, had to reconcile contradictory messages. Her education taught her the American way, but her family taught something else. "Growing up, I went to an all-white school where the ideal was tall and skinny," she reported. "I exercised and watched what I ate at school, but then at home I was encouraged to eat and eat."

She would then spend summers in Ecuador, where she was told, "You look like you're dying—you're too thin." She would eat a great deal while there. When she returned to the United States, an altogether opposite message awaited her: "If you want to be popular and attractive, you have to be thin." She became bulimic, which actually demonstrated the battles going on within. Eventually she went to work for a magazine, where the models on its pages became her feminine ideal.

Skin tone is another issue for some Hispanic-American women, who mentioned warnings from their mothers to avoid staying out in the sun or on the beach too long. One mother cautioned, "You'll look like a field worker." Another would say, "Don't surf too much, you're getting too dark." The latter mother kept her own hands covered and wore a big hat to protect her skin. She always told her daughter, "White is more beautiful."

CHINESE, VIETNAMESE, AND KOREAN

The ideal Chinese beauty is thin, small breasted, demure, and very feminine. A Chinese-American woman said, "The ideal beauty is skinny. And it is not a muscular-looking skinny. It's a very weak-looking thinness. Female beauty for the Chinese is very girlie: long hair, simple makeup, and very modest dress. It is never flashy and never has too much exposed skin."

There is a strong message about the passive role females should take. Comments by a Chinese-Vietnamese woman suggest the ideal is based on male insecurities. "Large women defy the ideal image in that they are threatening, since the men in our culture are pretty small themselves. There is a negative stereotype for larger women, who are seen as too aggressive and too independent—that which you are not supposed to be."

The ideal of beauty in the Korean culture has shifted, according to one Korean-American woman. "Traditionally a modest woman, represented by fair skin, a gentle and reserved manner, and who is not overtly attractive in body and face was considered beautiful. But there are signs of Westernization," she said.

Research shows Asian women have the highest proportion of individuals who value light skin. A Chinese-American woman noted, "Skin is preferred white rather than tan. The skin-whitening industry in Asia is big, and continues to grow as Asians are beginning to adopt Western ideals of beauty. They wear padded bras, and breast implants and eyelid surgery are the most popular plastic surgeries in Asia. The eyelid surgery creates a Western fold in the eye cover in order to create a more open eye and of course allow you to wear eye shadow."

AFRICAN AMERICAN

African-American women described attractiveness in terms of shapeliness, femininity, hips and buttocks, and the idea of "looking good."

Some descriptions of the ideal African-American woman include:

"She is curvy and full figured and classy."

"The ideal beauty is approximately a size 14 to 18. She's tall, has smooth skin, and can style her hair in a variety of ways. Her breasts are average size, about a 38 or 40B. She has a pear-shaped body."

"The African-American woman has very strong features that are head turners, with full lips, curvy hips, firm thighs, and long, slightly bow legs, tall and friendly with shoulder-length hair."

"African women are beautiful no matter what. . . . African women as a whole are happier with their bodies."

Such statements reflect the positive body image of many African-American women, yet there is also a negative side. Due to the influence of American culture, white physical features such as straight hair and light skin are valued.

Because one woman's great-grandmother was raped by a white man, her grandmother had very light skin and straight hair. So did her mother. This woman's own hair, however, was kinky. She remembers how her grandmother would braid it, openly voicing her disgust. "It hurts to braid your hair," she would say. "I never thought my grandchild would have black nappy hair." This woman has spent most of her adult life coming to terms with her body and her dark skin.

Another African-American woman commented on how freeing it was when black militant Angela Davis wore her hair natural in the sixties. "It was the first time I ever saw that," she says. "I felt that I could stop trying to control, change, straighten my hair, and let it be."

On the other hand, one middle-aged African-American woman received support for her dark skin. "My mother always said to me, 'The blacker the berry the sweeter the juice.' " This mother, who had a very positive body image, also told her, "I buy clothes to fit my body, not a fashion model's body."

CAUCASIAN

For Caucasians, who come from many different ethnic groups, the ideal beauty is almost always thin, and often blonde. In the workshop, a fourth generation Irish-American woman, thirty-three, spoke of the conflicts she experiences.

"The message for Irish women when I was growing up was that women have to be strong enough to work . . . on the farm along with their fathers, brothers, husbands, and sons. So the idea of being Twiggy is not part of the Irish female psyche.

"Since women work so hard in and out of the house, they remain quite trim yet solid, and would probably be considered stocky in America. Food was very important to Irish families, especially because there were times in Ireland when food was scarce. And they knew what it meant not to have food.

"Many Irish women are solid and strong. They do not concern

themselves with looking like Barbie because their energy remains focused on staying strong enough to wear their many hats throughout the day. Another example of their beauty can be seen in their chapped, dry hands from working on the farm, wrinkles from worrying about others, bags under their eyes from lack of sleep because they were busy doing dishes, laundry, and cleaning house.

"As hard as Irish women work for others, they are equally concerned with taking care of what is important to them, which is their love for their families and their integrity."

She admits feeling trapped wishing she were more Irish; that is, less focused on her physical appearance and more focused on showing her beauty through her heart and actions. "However, the American part of me is concerned with my hair and my makeup and is obsessing over my weight all the time."

Despite her conflict, however, her background is nourishing. Compare it to this observation by a thirty-nine-year-old woman, self-described as "from the hills of Kentucky": "The ideal beauty in my part of Appalachia is thin, blonde, and large breasted. She's sexy and Barbie dollish."

Another Caucasian woman described the female ideal she learned as "Tall, tan, busty, and blonde with blue eyes, long legs, and tight buttocks." Interestingly, maternal qualities revered in other cultures are often totally missing from the Caucasian women's feminine ideals.

WHAT MEN LIKE

Most heterosexual women in the workshop and in my research based their ideal body image on what men of their culture prefer. One woman noted that men in Cuba want light to dark skin; long, dark hair; large breasts; a tiny waist; and curvy, ample hips and thighs.

Appalachian men are infatuated by the Barbie doll image. According to the woman from Kentucky, "I think Barbie is considered ideal because of what I call the Appalachian male syndrome, where men want to be able to tell their women exactly what they can do and where. They feel they own their wives or girlfriends.

"They yearn for a wife or girlfriend who looks like Barbie but is Harriet Nelson at home. Women and young girls are captivated by the fact that men are so excited by this type, and they in turn try to mimic the image," she says.

Research with men indicates that African-American and Hispanic men prefer heavier female figures than do white men. This creates for these women a subculture in which heavier figures are acceptable.

A thirty-one-year-old African-American woman wrote, "Just from observing black women over the years, I noticed that we generally are a little bit thicker than white women. Black men seem to be attracted to women with a little extra padding. There is an old African-American saying that 'Nobody likes a bone but a dog.' As a black woman I don't want to be fat, but I don't want to be skinny either."

Other African-American women said:

"I've heard my uncles say forever, 'I like my women like the lobster—all the meat in the tail.' "

"In my early forties I married a man who loves my body type and makes me feel that I am sexy to him even though I am now a 16 to 18. I was a 14 to 16 when we got married."

"According to the teenage boys I grew up with, a girl with big legs, round buttocks, and ample breasts was the most desirable."

*   *   *

"I can remember when I was fifteen or sixteen and complaining to my mother that I hated my large legs and behind. She looked at me and said, 'Honey, that is your heritage. Your people are built that way and black men like that.' We were built to be able to bear children, work, and handle loving a black man. This body type shows off our heritage. We don't walk, we strut what God has given us with pride."

Over and over again it became apparent how crucial a positive male response is to a woman's body image and confidence, regardless of cultural background. Wrote a Caucasian woman, "I have a boyfriend who loves my body. He doesn't care that my boobs are tiny A-cups, especially when compared to my hips. He is unbelievably accepting. Actually, I've learned that most men are. I really think that women are far more critical of themselves and each other than men."

Someone else said, "My husband thinks I am beautiful, perfect, very sexy, and a most wonderful lover." Says another who is overweight, "My husband of twenty-four years always says that he loves me just as I am. He never makes a remark about my body."

A negative reaction, however, can shake a woman's world. An African-American social worker described how her husband, who had always been positive about her body, suddenly changed his preferences. For the first time, when she gained some weight, he urged her to lose it. Why the turnabout? She, a Ph.D., and her husband, a lawyer, were upwardly mobile. He spent more and more time with Caucasians, receiving more exposure to their preferences and attitudes. Increasingly he identified with the dominant culture. Even the magazines he read changed.

His reaction upset her tremendously. She felt he wanted her to look like white women in magazines, and she began to see herself differently. She felt less appealing. Although she told her husband, "This is ridiculous. I'm getting older. I've had three kids. I can't and I don't want to look like a white magazine model." Nevertheless, she had conversations with herself along the lines of, "I don't feel as good about myself. I'm not as athletic-looking as I used to be. I felt more attractive then."

That such an assertive woman should be so affected by her husband's response may seem surprising, yet a Korean-American woman echoes this reality. "There's no question that the popular images influence social expectations of what is considered beautiful in American culture. Moreover, such images deeply affect a woman's own expectations of how she should or wants to look. Despite the awareness of anorexia and the postfeminist era I've grown up with, there is still a rigid beauty ideal perpetuated by media images and the cult of celebrity. As a feminist I still feel the pressure." Many women would respond the same way.

THE ROLE OF RITUALS AND DANCES

Throughout history, whenever a conquering group wanted to crush the vanquished population, it would ban them from performing their old rituals, as well as speaking their own language. It was an effective technique, because it disconnected people from their key tools for maintaining personal balance and integration.

During the workshop, I asked the participants what ethnic rituals and celebrations taught them about the meaning of their bodies. Asian, African-American, Hispanic, and Muslim women talked about the nourishing power of the rituals they were taught. Yet as people assimilate, rituals from their culture of origin fade or are dropped entirely, which further encourages feelings of discontinuity.

A twenty-six-year-old woman from the Punjab region of India speaks fondly of the rituals and dances she has learned to celebrate the female body and mind. Her culture teaches her that she doesn't have to be thin to be beautiful. What matters are strength and character. She wrote, "The ideal Punjabi woman has beautiful almond-shaped eyes, full lips, and long, jet black hair. She is not thin. There is much poverty in India, so when a woman has some curves, people can tell she comes from money because she obviously has enough money to buy food to eat. She also has a great sense of self-esteem. The way people can identify this trait is in the way she walks. There are many songs and poems devoted to the way a Punjabi woman walks. A big part of the walk is having full hips that catch the eye when they sway. However, all the physical characteristics should also accompany an internal sense of strength."

She notes that the majority of Punjabi women are of the Sikh religion, where women have a history of being warriors. "There were stories told to us of women who fought in battles and were strong enough to fight right alongside the men three hundred years ago," she explains.

She mentioned a dance called Giddha, which was performed during festivals and in times of great joy, such as weddings and births. All the women of the village would get together in a circle and dance to verses. Every woman was accepted and wanted. "That same tradition continues here today when Indian women of every age get together and dance at weddings," she says.

Caucasians come from a whole spectrum of ethnic groups that have their own rituals. Sadly, however, the ritual mentioned by Caucasians was often dieting—a ritual that depletes, rather than enriches, you.

"What my aunts and I do at Christmas is discuss the newest diet. And who's gained and who's lost," said a workshop participant. She envied the women who talked about getting together, cooking recipes, and sharing stories. "I'd rather be doing what you do," she said.

Someone else wrote, "The only ethnic tradition I learned was dieting. . . . Since I was a child, my mother and aunts were concerned about my weight. We used to pray at night that I wouldn't wind up with my Aunt Karen's thighs. We didn't share ethnic dances. We suffered through aerobic classes to lose weight. There were no rich ethnic stories passed down—instead information about diets, low-fat recipes, and spas to go to in order to lose weight were shared. I can never remember feeling positive about my body, even as a child."

Another Caucasian said, "Once in a while I would buy *National Geographic* magazine and read with amazement that these strong tribal women were celebrated, adored, and showered with attention. There were different skin colors, shapes, sizes. They were photographed without makeup. They were beautiful. I wonder if my feelings about my body would have been more positive if I grew up with these pictures and danced in these tribal rituals."

Finally, one woman was a mournful witness to the Americanization of her culture's dancing tradition.

The workshop participant of Irish descent lamented the Americanization of Irish dancing, which is a tradition for both females and males. "It takes a lot of strength and endurance, as well as practice. Many Irish dancers are fit yet healthy-looking. Ironically, America has transformed the look of Irish dancing into more of a show, which is now female based, and the women are getting skinnier and skinnier. They wear lots of makeup and their clothes are tight and sexy, which is not traditional at all to Irish dancing. They have turned Irish dancing into just another form of entertainment."

THE ANDROGYNY FACTOR

African-American women in my workshop were the most likely to describe themselves with both masculine and feminine traits. Because their male ancestors were often slaves, part of the story they learned was, "You can't count on a man to be there. You have to support yourself and run a family. You have to be able to put food on the table and pay the bills." In a way, that has led them to become more independent and self-sufficient, qualities that traditionally are seen as masculine.

There's a connection between possessing androgynous traits and the more positive body image of African-American women. Research has found that gender-typed individuals—for example, women who are totally feminine—are more likely than non-gendered individuals to be influenced by appearance stereotypes.

If you feel, "I'm a woman. Therefore I can never get my hands dirty. I can never go out and kick a ball," you tend to be more at risk for body image problems and overconcerned about how you look. The ability of African-American women to express their masculine side seems to account for part of why they enjoy such a positive body image.

The experience of a Caucasian workshop participant illustrates what can happen when the masculine side is silent. A slim, soft-looking blonde, she arrived early for the morning walk on the second day of the workshop. To prepare her for photos that would be taken later for *O* magazine, a makeup artist went to work on her, applying cosmetics. She sat passively having her hair fixed and a scarf wound around her hair to add color. All made up, she proceeded to go on the group walk—and hated every minute of it. She kept her discontent to herself, however.

Hours later, during a discussion, she cried as she talked about how much the makeup experience had upset her. It reminded her of a time long ago when she'd regularly become what the world had wanted her to be. She'd followed the trends then. If girls had worn their hair down and curly, she'd done that, too. If models had worn blue eye shadow and mascara, that's what she'd worn. But she had changed, and she lived more authentically now. The makeup experience, which had sculpted her into someone she wasn't, had cast her back into an old role. She had even regressed into old behavior. Since the walk, she'd found herself comparing her appearance to other women's—something she hadn't done in a very long time. Passively allowing others to decide what was appropriate for her had thrown off her whole day.

A while later, she had a chance to express her anger at the experience in a unique and therapeutic way. That afternoon an African-American musician was leading a workshop to teach participants how to drum. When he arrived, he gave each of us a tall drum. First he taught the basics, explaining the different parts of the instrument and demonstrating how to hit it with your hands. Then we had a chance to develop our own beat, which the others could imitate. As the woman above pounded her drum, she felt wonderful. "I never tried this before," she explained, "and I thought, 'This will be awful, this is something men do out in the forest, yelling, screaming.'" But she made a surprising discovery. Although she enjoyed creating her own beat, what she loved best was banging that drum aggressively. It made her feel alive and full of energy. In drum class, this passive woman was no longer passive.

Before her setback earlier that day, she had been living her life more authentically, which had improved her body image and made her more attractive to men. She was in a healthy relationship with a man who loved her, and she was having the best sex of her life. Expressing her masculine side through drumming returned her to that healthy state.

TIPS FROM OTHER CULTURES
ON IMPROVING BODY IMAGE

The sweeping cultural changes over the last thirty years may have left us feeling disconnected from values and traditions that center us and help us feel secure. At a time when we yearn for meaning in our lives, we need to honor what is nourishing in our heritages of origin and what is positive in American culture in order to feel good about ourselves and create something uniquely our own. Here's how.

PICK THE BEST OF BOTH CULTURES

A twenty-nine-year-old Latina administrative assistant writes, "In my parents' culture I'm only seen as a married woman with three kids. A mother, that's who I am. To them it's okay to gain weight as you get older when you are a mother. But I'm not from Latin America. I work in a health spa where women are watching what they eat and exercising to stay in shape as they age. I don't want to have diabetes and heart disease during midlife like most of the women in my family."

Like many women, she feels a clash of cultures every day. But she doesn't have to choose one or the other. She can give voice to both parts of herself. Although she may not choose to follow the dietary habits of her Latino background on a day-to-day basis, she does love the gatherings and celebrations that revolve around food. "Food is a huge source of comfort in my family. We're very close and we celebrate every holiday together. We make tamales from 7 A.M. to 2 P.M. It's fun. Cooking, eating, laughing, the focal point is food."

Through therapy, a Hispanic woman in the workshop who became bulimic realized that she could create her own female ideal. She didn't have to have seven children, and breast-feed every one, as her mother and grandmother did. She could embrace what was maternal in her, yet also be someone who could make things happen in the world. She could accept that she had a rounder bottom than she used to, but she could also exercise to stay in shape.

Other groups can make similar choices. If your family has focused on diets, you can encourage female relatives to get out of the cage by banning diet discussions, and asking each other instead about your kids, your jobs, your opinions, and your passions.

DEVELOP THE MASCULINE PART OF YOU

To achieve a positive body image, it is important that women develop both the masculine and feminine aspects of themselves. Women who do, seem to better resist the culture's female ideal—and form their own.

The woman in the drumming story felt powerful when she expressed her masculine side. It pulled her out of the depression she was feeling. "I didn't care how I looked when I was drumming," she told the group, grinning. "By the time I was done, makeup was all over my face, and I was sweating and smelled from perspiration. But it didn't matter."

Other voices confirm the joy of being connected to their masculinity.

A Chinese-Vietnamese woman found it very hard to grow up being the biggest girl in class. "I learned to have a strong personality that can overcome any opposition," she said. "My peers, family members, and people on the street constantly reminded me that I was big—like a boy. They did not mention fat in most cases, but they would say, 'My goodness, you're a big Asian girl.' I've learned to answer them with, 'Big deal. Not one person is perfect. I would appreciate it if you would accept me for who I am.' "

She added, "Eleanor Roosevelt said that no one can make you feel inferior without your consent. I truly feel I'm the only person who can control how I feel about my body." She loves her body and all its "unfeminine" strength.

A thirty-four-year-old woman of French-Portuguese descent has learned to embrace her masculine side by admiring female athletes. "Seeing their strong, healthy bodies helps me better accept my own natural tendency toward masculinity. I have been able to make some progress in overcoming my negative beliefs about my body by focusing on my athleticism. I recognize the variety of body types as part of God's plan, and that my body shape has nothing to do with my value as a human being. I focus on strength, not appearance. I work on strengthening my body and feel good when I am able to."

Another Caucasian woman feels pride in her strength, noting, "Some of my weight gain is due to muscle strength, as I am able to do more physically than a lot of women who weigh less. I have proven that to myself and others many times both in and out of the military, by being able to move heavy equipment that other women can't. Some men value having a strong female, more than they do having an attractive female. A reliable female who can manage on her own without having every tough task wait until a male is available is one of the things that males like. That is something that I was taught by my relatives as I was growing up, and it has stayed with me."

VALUE THE RITUALS AND CELEBRATIONS OF YOUR HERITAGE

Don't abandon your own culture and history. Rituals have meaning and renew our spirit. If we are to get past our present cultural emptiness and tendency toward addictions, including food addictions, we need to incorporate meaningful rituals in our lives not only to balance and mobilize ourselves—but to anchor our children as well.

Ironically, *The New York Times* reports that in New Orleans, Vietnamese youth who are least assimilated—who speak the language at home and with friends, celebrate ethnic holidays, and attend church with family—tend to be the achievers. Delinquent Vietnamese adolescents are more likely to be the most Americanized, shunning their culture of origin and idolizing rock stars.[1] It is not surprising. Connection with their own culture gives youngsters a more solid sense of self so that they don't have to turn to gangs for identity, rules, and language.

Whatever our background, we give our children a gift by continuing to celebrate the holidays we or our parents grew up with. But sometimes we need to create new rituals in our lives because we move so much more than we used to, and lose traditional supports.

You can be creative in reconciling the realities of modern life with rituals that are important to you, as a recently divorced woman in one of my groups realized. In the past, she, her husband, and children celebrated Easter together. They would color eggs and hide Easter baskets, and she would invite her husband's relatives, who were the only family that lived nearby, for Easter dinner. Since that arrangement was not possible after the divorce, she decided to try something different. For the first time, she took her two children on vacation all by herself. The trip to Florida took place during the kids' spring school break. Toward the end of the vacation, she jokingly mentioned to her kids, "We'll be flying back on Easter Sunday, so there won't be any Easter baskets or Easter dinner this year."

As the family drove home from the airport on Easter Sunday, her son inquired, "Mom, can't we pretend that next Sunday is Easter?" Life was changing for these children and there was a certain security for them in knowing that they could maintain this holiday. Even though they were thirteen and fifteen, and didn't believe in the Easter bunny anymore, they both loved Easter baskets filled with special chocolates, marshmallow bunnies, and other goodies. They were accustomed to Easter dinner. Although they loved the new ritual of going on vacation, they wanted and needed the old tradition, as well.

There is something about the repetition in rituals that soothes us, makes us feel safe, and tells us who we are. In this case Easter says, "We are Christian, and this is part of our story. These are the smells and colors of our foods."

Rituals don't only have to focus on eating. A ritual of dressing nourished a Korean-American woman. "Asian cultures vary quite a bit, but several east Asian traditional dresses serve to actually cover up the woman's body while also connoting femininity either through sensuous fabric or through the special ritual of getting dressed. The Korean dress is full, flowing, and yet also gave me a sense of womanhood and beauty that I think was distinctly Asian rather than American," she said.

She was referring to the art of dressing, which all of us can enjoy in our way. Wouldn't it be wonderful to put time aside before going out on a weekend night to dress in a leisurely fashion—to have a cup of tea, smooth lotion on your body, and enjoy the sensuous fabrics of the clothing you've chosen. How relaxing and sensual it can be to experience the beauty of your body in that way.

EXPLORE OTHER CULTURES

To remind yourself that there is more to life than just American culture, why not try something from another ethnic background? As Stacy, a forty-year-old career woman with two young children discovered, the experience can change you in very positive ways. Stacy, who participated in one of my groups, described how frumpy and unattractive she felt. She had gained thirty pounds since her pregnancies and overate at most meals. The image she had of her body was one that was shapeless and asexual. She joked that pretty soon she'd be buying muumuus like her mother and aunts wore.

However, a remark by another woman in the group led her on another path. The woman mentioned that she had recently started taking belly dancing lessons. She loved the new way she was moving her body, especially her hips. She couldn't remember moving that way since her twenties.

Intrigued by what she'd heard, Stacy decided to take belly dancing lessons, too. She loved the sensuous fabrics, costumes, and the rhythms of the music. The teacher encouraged students to explore their sensuality and the different ways their bodies could move, in a way that Stacy's mother was never able to. Stacy bought CDs of some of the music played in class to enjoy at home. Although her husband thought she had gone off the deep end, Stacy experienced sheer joy in her new movement. She found herself overeating less and motivated to exercise. She reported feeling as if she had a shape, and she no longer saw herself as a big "box."

DO A REALITY CHECK ON WHAT MEN LIKE

We don't want partners to dictate how we look. But at the same time, we want to be attractive to the person we're attracted to. Research shows that African-American women are more accurate than other groups about what their men consider attractive in females—ample hips, buttocks, and breasts. This is important, since a partner's positive response to her body is crucially important to a woman, regardless of ethnic group. If your man likes the way you look and you know it, you're likely to have a good body image no matter what your weight or shape or skin tone.

The rest of us need to talk more to men about what they find appealing. What can you say to a man to find out? Something like, "I notice you tend to like women who are curvy." Or, "What initially attracted you to me?"

You can also talk about what you as a woman find sexually attractive about your partner, as in, "I love warm, compassionate men with sexy eyes" or "I love men who make me laugh."

Then listen to the feedback you get. I believe women will find that most men, at the very least, want curves, not stick-thin women.

Men can help women with their body image, but they need to be more aware of what they say. Let men know that their words can hurt you. Speak up and tell them, "You're important to me, and what you say affects how I feel."

FIND A SUPPORTIVE PARTNER AND COMMUNITY AND REALIZE YOUR SPIRITUALITY

A bulimic woman ended her relationship with a boyfriend who wanted her to be skinny. Instead, she found a man who liked rounded women. An African-American woman overcame a negative body image this way: "I continually reinforced to myself that looks are not the be-all and end-all of a person. I also surround myself with people who feel the same way so we can reinforce this notion and help each other stay positive and focused on what's really important in life."

A middle-aged African-American woman improved her body image by refusing to read or support magazines that fail to celebrate the diversity of true beauty. "By only surrounding myself with photos and paintings of more diverse women. By realizing that every woman has her own unique loveliness, and the more diverse from the standard the more beautiful to me. By simply getting older and more spiritual, and realizing that the Creator has made all women beautiful no matter what type, color, age."

A thirty-one-year-old Korean-American commented, "Now I

am content. I attribute it to my peace of mind and my faith and spirituality. Things such as looks become very trivial where matters of faith and soul and heart are concerned. I'm married now with twin boys. Life is definitely much more meaningful and more defined by what is unseen than what is seen. When I see my face in the mirror, I see my soul."

A twenty-eight-year-old Caucasian woman wrote, "I moved close to the mountains and it's very healthy for me. Just being outdoors, hiking, and enjoying the scenery is fun and promotes fitness. I forget about my weight, which I've been obsessed with all my life, because I'm having too much fun hiking, walking, and watching the birds."

HAVE A DIVERSE GROUP OF FRIENDS

Accepting other people and appreciating cultural differences goes together with accepting yourself. A Caucasian woman whose father was a teacher working with migrant workers grew up in a house filled with people of different sizes, shapes, ethnic groups, and skin colors.

"At my house we listened to black music," she recalled. "I learned dances that emphasized and glamorized large hips. I loved how the workers talked about ideas, not about how people looked. I didn't watch much TV. Too much was going on at home. For the most part I accepted my body. I was taught to enjoy the different cultures, diverse foods, different shapes and weights. I would rather pick up a copy of *National Geographic* than a fashion magazine."

It undoubtedly helped this girl with her body image to see that big hips were appreciated, rather than hidden under baggy clothes as something shameful.

Not all of us have had such exposure to people of other cultures, but you can be deliberate about reaching out to individuals in various ethnic groups in the workplace and the community. It's likely to enrich your life.

HONOR THE SEASONS OF YOUR WOMANHOOD

Maternal qualities formed the ideal in the Navajo culture, according to a Native-American woman. "Being a woman and being beautiful focused on mother earth, mothers, mother nature. This includes broad, childbearing hips, a very womanly figure, the hourglass shape."

She goes on to say, "Native-American women, or at least in my specific case, were taught to absolutely celebrate our role as life givers and maternal life forces. We are honored and respected. Our mother's clan is the dominant one. So when we are asked about our heritage and clans, we always identify ourselves with our mother's clan."

The Native-American attitude toward aging women is very positive as well. Said another Native American, "American-Indian women grow more beautiful with age. When my mother died, people remarked that she grew more beautiful with each passing year."

All women can take a lesson from Navajo beliefs and honor and respect every aspect of womanhood.

DEVELOP AN INTERNAL LOCUS OF CONTROL

An internal locus of control is essential for a positive body image. When women try to sculpt their bodies into the dominant culture's ideal, they feel inauthentic, self-conscious, and negative about their appearance.

A forty-three-year-old Asian-Indian woman overcame negative feelings about her body by switching the focus to what's important to her, instead of trying to please the rest of the world. She said, "I believe God has a mission for me, and thin is not it. I look at Gandhi, Martin Luther King, and how they used their lives for the betterment of society, and I now choose to lead my life in their shadow. In spite of my size 14, I have great friends and lovers."

SIX POINTS ABOUT ETHNICITY AND BODY IMAGE

Here are important highlights from research and from workshops I've led:

1. Body image is not just about weight and shape, which is more the focus of Caucasian women. For women of color, it's also about skin tone, hair, and personal style.

2. Standards of attractiveness do vary across cultures, and it's recognized now that preoccupation with thinness among women in the United States isn't totally mirrored within ethnic minority populations. However, very overweight individuals in almost all ethnic groups usually aspire to weight loss.[2]

3. Immigrant mothers and grandmothers exaggerated feminine stereotypes because they wanted their daughters to carry on their cultural traditions—which they feared would disappear under the influence of the dominant culture.

4. Most research shows that both Caucasians and Hispanics show the most weight-related disturbance, Asians and African Americans the least. Studies of African-American women clearly indicate a lesser preoccupation with achieving a slender body, and their body image is strongly influenced by consideration of their shape as well as their weight. Body size isn't necessarily central to the perception of one's self as attractive.

   As Hispanics become more assimilated, they seem to

have more conflict about appearance. In my research on adolescents, Hispanic girls were most likely to be thinking about plastic surgery such as liposuction and breast augmentation. Hispanic women and Caucasians talked about wanting bigger breasts, but that wasn't as much an issue for Asian and African-American girls. That also fits the research. However, I believe that this is beginning to change as Asian women become more Americanized.

5. In the workshop, not one of the women mentioned experiencing racism based on her physical appearance except within her family of origin. Although that experience might be limited to participants, it might also indicate that things are changing.

6. Women in the workshop talked about seeing more ethnically diverse models these days, although these models all have the same thin shape. The next step would be diverse bodies, as well. An African-American woman mentioned celebrities like Leslie Uggams and Whoopi Goldberg as aiding acceptance of dark skin.

It is important we move away from treating each ethnic group as a monolithic whole and look at factors that influence body image satisfaction or dissatisfaction. We know, for example, that social class affects women's body image perception. Recent research shows that both white and black women of higher socioeconomic status feel pressure to be thin.

Other issues, such as the individual's attitude toward her own socio-racial group, should be considered, as well. In one study, African-American women who were unhappy with their skin color tended to have more negative body images than those who were not. Interracial contact, the amount of exposure a person has to the dominant culture, also warrants attention. To what extent have these women internalized the dominant society's definition of beauty? And who are these women comparing themselves to? For instance, if African-American women compare themselves to other African-American women, they will probably have a more positive body image than if they compare themselves to white or Asian women. Large buttocks and hips are seen as beautiful in African-American women, but not in Asian or white females.

We need to move beyond seeing each ethnic group as separate and self-contained. Globalization has changed things, and our thinking must change, too.

9

STRUT YOUR STUFF

Our deepest fear is that we are powerful beyond measure. It
is our light not our darkness that most frightens us. We ask
ourselves, "Who am I to be brilliant, gorgeous, talented, fab-
ulous?" Actually who are you not to be? You are a child of
God. Your playing small does not serve the world.
                                                    Marianne Williamson,
                                                    A Return to Love

A group of women eat breakfast together in the restaurant of a
Palm Springs hotel as their husbands attend meetings in the conference center. They sit in rapt attention as one of them, a mother
of three and a grandmother, describes her experience of passing
fifty. "It was the most emancipating experience of my life," she
says. "At forty-nine I was a little depressed about getting older,
but at fifty I didn't have to explain my kids' behavior or choices
anymore. I didn't care what others said about me. It was 'I'm
okay, and if you don't like me, it's your problem.'

"I felt all right about my failures and knew that there were a lot
of things I could do with the rest of my life. The first thing I
wanted to do was confront my fears. I was always terrified of
heights, so I went up in a balloon. After that, I took a helicopter
ride over the Matterhorn. There's more to life than fifty."

Facing down your demons is one of many ways to liberate

yourself as you get older. The years after menopause can become an era of creativity and growth, dubbed "postmenopausal zest" by the late anthropologist Margaret Mead. Are you ready to set the stage to strut your stuff?

STOP TRYING TO BE PERFECT

I first met Sally, fifty-one, a full-time homemaker who lives in Memphis, at a workshop several years ago, and she has kept in touch with me. One day she called to describe her weeklong vacation in Cancun, Mexico, with her stockbroker husband and two teenage sons. Sally is someone who feels that she should look her best at all times. Ordinarily, she never goes into the ocean, although she knows how to swim. When her family asks her to join them in the water, her response is always, "I don't want my hair to get messed." Or, "I don't want to get too dirty." Or, "I don't want the sand on me." This time, however, was different.

"I just decided to do it," she told me. "Big waves were rolling in, and my husband and kids were having a ball, so I went in." She got knocked over in the surf, jumped around all afternoon, and felt like a kid again. Exhausted afterward, she went back to the room. Her husband handed her a beer, which tasted great. Then she took a nap. When the family went out for pizza later, everyone talked about the waves. "I was right in there," she bragged, obviously pleased with herself.

It sounded like a wonderful time, yet I quickly detected something negative in her tone. After gentle prodding, she admitted feeling ambivalent about her no-holds-barred, messy play. At her age, she thought it was somehow inappropriate.

Like many midlife women I see, Sally got her pleasure from trying to be perfect, which often left her standing on the sidelines, distanced from others. She was actually a very lonely person, although you wouldn't know that if you met her. She was usually surrounded by her family or friends. But her source of good feelings about herself came from other people telling her, "You never have a hair out of place." Or, "You never forget a detail." Or, "This dinner party is a dream right down to the flowers." She didn't derive pleasure from closeness with people, however. She had no soul mates in whom to confide intimate aspects of herself. She didn't share feelings of compassion and never experienced the inner glow which comes from that. Our work together focused on helping her trade in the good feelings she got from being perfectly dressed, the perfect hostess, the perfect organizer—and feeling superior to everybody—for the joy that comes from being connected. That involved moving out of the cage where she simply watched what others were doing, to becoming an active and freer participant in life.

"Hold on to that wonderful way you felt sloshing around in the water," I urged her. "After a wave knocked you down, your son helped you up; then you helped him up. You and your husband were giggling. At a time like that no one cares whether your mascara is running. Maybe you're ready to join the rest of the crew and get closer."

Her son had said, "Hey, Mom, we might even start taking you to football games." I told her, "If you had a daughter, those words would have been, 'I feel closer to you.' Guys don't say that, but I bet it was freeing for your boys to see your hair all wet and tangled."

Why do many women feel the need to be perfect? Sometimes we feel so bad about ourselves that we think it is the only way to be acceptable. Or we were criticized so much when we were growing up that we feel we have to be flawless to head off attack. Sally's perfectionism traced back to her mother, who always found fault with her. Even though her mom died years ago, her voice lived on in Sally.

Sally's mother's influence wasn't all bad. She did teach her good things about mothering, keeping a household together, and listening to people. Sally's father had been an alcoholic who couldn't hold a job. Her mother had had to work to support the family. She taught Sally how to take care of herself and find an ambitious, successful man. She showed her what a better life would be. Even though there wasn't much money, she dressed Sally up at Easter with lovely clothes. She took her to tea, and taught her how to act like a lady. She talked to her about all the things she would love to do herself if she wasn't working. Yet her mother, who probably felt frustrated, constantly told her that she had to look and act perfect.

At the beach, Sally had actually commented, "I'm such a mess, I look like an alcoholic." I told her, "I think that's your mother's voice of disapproval. I think she believed that if somehow she could make you perfect you'd have a better life than hers. But that's not what's made your life better. You have to let go of that." Sally had to separate her mother's voice from her own.

Does Sally's story resonate with you? Do you set up perfectionist standards for yourself to maintain a sense of control and ward off loneliness? If so, you need to let go. Imagine putting your worries in a balloon each night and releasing them. Watch them fly away, and slowly relax as you realize they are gone. Then start using your energy the next day to change the things in your life that you do have control over, such as taking good care of yourself and developing closer relationships with others.

REVISE YOUR CONCEPT OF MISTAKES

Midlife is about growth and change. You can't grow when you're always trying to be perfect, because growth involves taking healthy risks and sometimes making mistakes.

Over and over in the Olympics, even ice-skating finalists stumble or fall as they execute jumps and other difficult movements. How do they react? They get up and continue seamlessly, leaving their mistakes behind. I remember a TV commentator asking one skater, "What were you thinking during your performance as you lay on the ice after your fall?" She answered, "That I have to get up, period."

The next time you fall, perhaps by bingeing at breakfast, don't waste energy beating yourself up. And don't say, "I blew it. I might as well overeat all day and start over tomorrow." Instead say, "I blew it. I am going to brush my teeth and start over at lunch and eat healthy." If you skip exercise for a week due to a work crisis, return to your normal workout routine the next week. Recovery is not about perfection. It's about quickly getting back on track, period.

When you get off track in other areas of your life, move ahead in the same way. Picture yourself in the car as the kids squabble in the backseat. Losing your temper, you yell at them, and maybe you even wind up running a red light and getting a traffic ticket. Instead of berating yourself and feeling bad or resentful, have a different dialogue with yourself. Insist, "It's done. I'm not going to obsess about it." Or reframe the "failure," focusing on how far you've come, with self-talk such as, "Boy, have I grown. Ten years ago this incident would have escalated and made me crazy for a week."

When you accept that mistakes are learning experiences that are part of being human, and you take them in your stride, you open yourself up to life. Amazing things can happen when and where you least expect them. A former patient who has come to terms with her own perfectionism after years of struggle described the following incident.

She and her husband went out to a local mall for a sushi dinner one night. As they pulled into the parking lot, she opened the car door to get out and narrowly missed hitting the side of a car that had just parked in an adjacent spot. The driver, who was headed to the same restaurant with his wife, growled at her, "You really ought to watch what you're doing. You almost scraped up my car." Instead of feeling shamed and embarrassed at her near mistake, she calmly explained, "I was distracted and didn't pay attention. But your car is fine. No harm done." Smiling at his continued scowl, and chuckling to herself about men and their cars, she then held out her hand and proposed, "Truce?"

The implication that people make mistakes was very freeing and disarmed the driver. As a result, a bit of an adventure followed. She recognized the man's wife as a friend of a friend, and the two couples wound up sharing a table at the restaurant. Discovering a lot in common, they had a great time talking over drinks. "Then from out of the blue, the husband suddenly looked me in the eye and said with admiration, 'How is it that you are so alive?' I felt so incredibly flattered. And he was right. I was alive," she remembers.

His response had nothing to do with her appearance. There were several attractive women in the restaurant. It was her vitality and spirit that made her so appealing. And that's what midlife can be about. Women have grown enough and become wise enough to accept, and even embrace, the fact that they are not, and will never be, perfect. They can feel entitled to make mistakes like everyone else, then own them and move on. When they do, they become very attractive to other people.

Revising their concepts of mistakes has freed up many women in my midlife workshops. One participant recounted a disastrous dinner party she hosted for close friends. She had decided to try a new chicken recipe, which bombed. In the past she would have obsessed, "Why did I have to experiment with a new dish? I should have stayed with a sure thing." But the inedible chicken actually made the evening, as the laughs continued all night.

Says the hostess, "We ate lots of salad and rice to fill ourselves up. No one left hungry, and we had a hilarious time because everyone let their hair down." Chances are she particularly endeared herself to her female guests, who could now feel they didn't have to be Martha Stewart either.

TAKE A NEW VIEW OF ACTING YOUR AGE

Part of allowing yourself to be imperfect involves changing the skewed view you may have of how you're supposed to be at your age. Many of us see the way our mothers and aunts acted and believe we must behave the same. It isn't so. Being alive is ageless. I remember the time I took my ten-year-old daughter Jennifer to Chicago for a mother-daughter weekend to shop for clothes before the start of the school year. Jennifer, who wants to be a designer someday, loves fashion. We bought lots of cute stuff for her in some offbeat stores, and she wanted to immediately wear some of her purchases. "Let's do it," I agreed.

Off we went out to lunch, and as we waited on line for a table, in walked a striking older woman. Although lines etched her face and neck, there was something very sensuous about her. Smoky eye shadow accented sexy blue eyes. She wore artsy, dangling earrings and a form-fitting outfit with a bohemian flair. Admiring the way Jennifer had accessorized herself, she asked, "Where did you get the great scarf and boots?" Jennifer returned the compliment with, "I love *your* clothes. I think you have a lot of the *p* factor—pizzazz."

As the woman burst out laughing, you could feel her energy. It seemed that two soul mates had made contact for a brief time.

Do you have pizzazz? Sally, who is very attractive, doesn't have it, but she could. She had it on the beach when she let herself go. Interestingly, she told me, "You know my husband and I made love that night in a way that we haven't in a long time. It was passionate and wonderful." I think he was excited by her letting go, and she felt excited herself.

She had also lamented that the day after her romp in the surf, her entire body felt sore. "I used to be able to jump around in the water easily," she said, "but this time I felt so wiped out that I slept for three hours afterward. What's wrong with me? Now I really feel like an older woman."

I assured her that there was nothing wrong with her. "That physical exhaustion from being in the ocean is a great feeling. It speaks to your body feeling energy—and now it needs to rest. You're on vacation having a ball with your family. Everyone loved joking with you. You don't sound old. You sound like someone letting go of acting old."

I have a group of career-oriented friends aged forty-six to fifty-two, whom I treasure because we break the rules together. We're all very supportive of taking risks that move us out of the cage. We recently met at someone's home to celebrate three birthdays at once. We chipped in, and one woman, a personal shopper, bought the presents—nightgowns that fit each person's personality.

When the first woman, who is heavy, opened her gift, she found a flowing style in an African motif. I remarked that when my mother got a present, she would jump up, run into the bathroom to change, and model it. It made the giver feel so good because her present made my mom so happy. All three women then decided to model their nightgowns. They wore them for the rest of the night.

When the husband of our hostess came downstairs, he found us laughing and talking all at once, and he saw three women in nightgowns. Awed by the scene, and our energy, he quipped, "Wow, this is a group of wild women." And he was right. It was just the sort of fun experience that I need as much as anyone else.

I get so involved in my work that I stop playing sometimes. It's important to deliberately put yourself with others and let loose.

Who are the people who inhibit you from letting go, being playful, and having fun? Do you know women with whom you can break the rules? Do you make it a point to get together? If such people are missing in your life, isn't it time to look around for likely candidates?

DARE TO GO FOR IT

We also need to reexamine our attitudes toward aggression. In order to do so, I often ask women to participate in this exercise. I tell them, "I want you to sit in a circle." I then put a piece of paper in the center.

"If you are being honest, you want all of the talking time. When I clap my hands, go after this one piece of paper the way you normally do when you need or want something in life. The percentage of talking time you get will be based on the percentage of paper you grab. If you get forty percent of the paper, you get forty percent of the time to talk." I clap my hands, and they all grab.

Then I say, "Close your eyes. I want you to notice whether your body feels or looks any different to you. Does it feel more tense? More relaxed? Does it feel fat? Or feel large, or small? Do certain parts, such as your feet, feel really big?"

Something fascinating happens every time. When women come away with a large piece of paper, they say things like, "I feel like large Marge. I'm greedy. I got most of the paper, but I feel people in the group are pissed off at me. They think, 'Boy, is she aggressive.'" Or someone will say, "For a minute I felt great, like 'I want it.' But after I went and got it and looked around the group, I felt bad because some members didn't get any paper at all. So I started breaking off pieces and giving them out. I felt better, but I also felt kind of ripped off."

I then ask them to repeat the exercise, instructing this time, "You have to do something different. If you weren't aggressive before, you have to be aggressive now. If you were aggressive before, be passive now."

I use this exercise to help midlife women identify and understand the concept of positive aggression, which is a source of life and growth. Aggression is present in all of us, from the time we are born. D. W. Winnicott[1] explains that a baby's aggression allows for curiosity to happen and for the baby to move out into the world and begin to explore it. It permits the child to develop an identity separate from the mother and establish a firm sense of self. If that does not occur, the child develops what Winnicott calls the false self. This happens to many women. They learn to please others, and they live separately from their true selves. They don't know what they need or hunger for. And if they do, they don't feel entitled to ask for it. They fear a negative response when they go after what they want.

Positive or creative aggression allows us an outlet through which we can express anger and take the initiative. As women, however, we learn to suppress aggression out of fear that we will be labeled unfeminine. The result can be seen in the statistics on depression in women: Twice as many women seek treatment for depression as men, and married women have higher rates of mental illness than married men.

Gender-typed individuals—women who allow themselves to express only their feminine characteristics—are more likely than nongendered individuals to be influenced by appearance stereotypes. To improve body image and self-esteem in midlife, it is crucial to express both the more traditional female parts of yourself and the male parts of yourself. It's important to be as comfortable going after what you want in a direct, effective way as it is to be able to put your own needs aside and help and nurture others.

What were you taught about aggressive women? Take a sheet

of paper and make a list of what comes to mind, such as, "Aggressive women are bitches." Or, "Aggressive women are like men." Then get out of the cage and do the exercise differently. Think of aggressive, successful women you admire to help you write down positive statements, such as "Aggressive women are smart." Or, "Aggressive women get the job done." Or, "Aggressive women help others effectively." This exercise can help you begin to think in a new way.

We are rarely taught to test the limits of our aggression—to play with it—as men do in sports. They go out, compete, bang themselves up, fall on their faces, and learn from it. Lawyers and politicians fight and then go have a beer together.

Even today smart women often don't feel the right to act aggressively. When they do, their appetite for achievement and success often leaves them feeling vulnerable. Many fear it will lead to the loss of personal relationships, and sometimes the struggle is expressed in their relationship with food.

I worked on this issue with Maureen, a fifty-five-year-old real estate executive who was wed for the second time. Very smart and accomplished, Maureen was more aggressive about her career than her friends and her husband were about theirs. She was also obsessed with dieting, although she was only a few pounds overweight. Her appetite for food and her appetite for success were definitely connected.

Maureen, who had just been promoted, knew that she was good at what she did and that others recognized her ability. She hoped to move to the top of her company. Yet she worried that taking achievement too far could ruin her personal life. Because her women friends were less successful than she, there were few of them she could talk to about the good things that kept happening to her at work. There's a certain comfort level women have with each other when they talk about their kids and college, planning a wedding or vacation, or lamenting a daughter's choice of boyfriend. That comfort often disappears when the topic changes to a great business deal or a promotion to an important position.

Maureen sensed, too, that her husband felt threatened. "I've got an idea for a new project that will really grow this outfit. I get all excited about it, and realize that I have power to influence the direction of the company. But when I discuss the idea with Bob, I think he's uncomfortable about it. I've got all this energy and excitement, but I don't have people to share it with," she complained.

As a result, Maureen felt that she had to keep her aggression underground. She acted on it instead by scrutinizing every calorie she ate. When she dined at a restaurant, she wanted to know the ingredients in every dish. If she couldn't keep her appetite for aggression in check, she could at least control her appetite for food.

Chinese women practiced footbinding, Victorian women laced themselves into corsets, and many of our mothers wore girdles. Contemporary women still go to extremes. They may have taken off the girdles their mothers wore, but they haven't discarded the "girdle mentality." Women's appetites, whether for food, power, or control, often leave them feeling exposed. Dieting can be a way to regain control and appear to be less voracious.

I worked with Maureen to explore issues of taking up space with her competency and creativity, using the image of a girdle that was constricting her. Gradually she began to realize, "My mother wore girdles and I always thought to myself, 'How ridiculous that she would wear those things to shape her body.' I thought I took the girdle off. Yet here I am weighing myself every day and analyzing everything I eat to keep myself in line. This is soaking up too much energy and time."

We were then able to explore questions such as, "Are you allowed to take the girdle off and free up your body, your ideas, and your talent?"

In cases such as Maureen's, I also meet with couples together to try to work out relationship solutions. (The same procedure would apply to same-sex couples.) The first step is to reassure the husband. I've found that some insecure men fear that a wife will leave if she becomes too successful or influential. Although Maureen's husband headed his own law practice, he wasn't the standout star that she was. He needed to hear her say, "No matter how far up the ladder I go, I will love you. I won't leave you."

Before we met together, however, I had to make sure Maureen did intend to stay in this marriage. I asked her privately, "Do you have any fears about meeting other men? You're going to be working with smart new people. You'll be traveling. Could it lead to an affair with someone else?"

She assured me, "No. I'm in my fifties; this is my second marriage. My children are grown. This is a good guy. I love him. I want to grow old with him. I have no interest in other men." Armed with this information, I could comfortably pose the same question in a joint session with him, and her answer could reassure him.

Next I could work on enlisting his support for her. But she had to contribute by being direct about what she needed from him. She needed him to listen to her ideas and show interest in her career, because that was an important part of who she was. He got the message and became a staunch supporter for her.

I talked with her, too, about learning to applaud herself when she got a promotion, rather than being dependent on others' reactions. She had to be able to tell herself, "I set goals and worked hard. I got coached. I read books. And because of my actions I got the job." Inner applause is an invaluable tool for mental health in general.

It is also important to have one or two friends who are more like you. Just recently a friend of mine left a message on my voice mail. "Ann, you won't believe this. I just got asked to be on a TV show. You're one of the few people I can tell." She's an educator who is very successful. She's written an important book and is being interviewed by the media. Her friends aren't that responsive to her triumphs because their worries and concerns are different from hers. However, I can say, "Good for you. Let me know when the show airs. I'll try to watch it." She does the same for me. In addition to being excited for each other, we're able to coach each other. She might ask, "What are some sound bites you can suggest? I'm too nervous to think of anything." And I can help her.

To strike up friendships with other women who share professional interests and concerns, you can join the boards of arts, philanthropic, or community organizations where you're likely to find others at a level similar to yours. You can also join professional groups in your field.

Allow yourself to be energetic, enterprising, bold, and aggressive—whether you are striving for a partnership in your firm or a seat on the town board or the presidency of the PTA. You deserve to achieve. By midlife you have acquired the wisdom of life experience. It's time to see yourself as a mentor and leader. Get outside the cage, go after what you want, and find new pathways for yourself and the women around you. Picture yourself thirty or forty years from now. Are you going to feel despair because so much of your life was defined by fear, rather than by choices you made?

DEVELOP MANY SOURCES OF SELF-ESTEEM

If you believe that your total value as a person hinges on how you look, you're going to have a hard time feeling good about yourself as you get older. But there are other options. As a midlife workshop participant once explained, "Focusing on the great job I did raising my children, the skills I've developed in sports, and my close relationships has really helped me to improve my body image." Curiosity, a spiritual life, and pursuit of learning can also be rich sources of self-esteem, which the aging of the body will never diminish.

For Bonnie, fifty-five, an effervescent wife and mother of three grown sons, finding meaningful work has been key in helping her develop self-esteem. Bonnie is someone who was never quite able to find a career niche—until now. Flitting from one thing to another, she did everything from selling insurance to managing an office. In each career she tried, she didn't stay long enough to get established because none of her choices felt right. Then she happened to attend a charity event, where she met a woman who was a career coach. As the coach described her work, Bonnie grew fascinated. A week later, she contacted the woman, who lived in another part of the country. Following her advice, Bonnie enrolled in a comprehensive training program. She has now started her own career-coaching practice.

"I found my true passion," says Bonnie. "Coaching is totally in sync with my values and needs. I have an uncommon ability to teach and inspire people and help them to reach their personal goals. My own coach helped me become who I am. I realized that I need approval and respect, which I didn't get in the other careers I tried. I gained confidence and stopped putting up with energy drainers in my life. Now I can fly. I can give to others because my needs are taken care of every day."

Bonnie's needs include losing weight and leading a balanced life. She has been extremely overweight for years. Now, however, she's determined to get healthy and take the weight off. As her self-esteem increases, her life takes on definition, and eventually so does her body.

Children and grandchildren can also bring joy, balance, and increased self-esteem to your life. I remember a summer night when my husband was working late and my two older children were out with friends. I took my two little ones, then eight and ten, out to eat and then to browse a local art supply store. "Let's see what they have on sale," I suggested. As we looked around, we found a beginner's watercolor kit that looked interesting, but both children preferred to pick out their own paints and brushes. I decided to buy the watercolor set for myself.

We came home, and since it was a wonderful night, we sat outside. I put on some soft classical music, and we all painted. When my son looked at what we produced, he proclaimed, "This is awesome. I think we should start an art gallery and sell them." Laughing, I realized that I really do enjoy painting. It makes me feel good.

Later, the kids went upstairs. My son took out an oak guitar we have, and my daughter grabbed a microphone. They improvised a mini rock band and created comedy skits. When my husband got home, tired and worried about his ill father, the children performed to cheer him up. In no time, they had him in hysterics.

It's so important to enjoy your children and grandchildren as you get older—or, if you don't have children, enjoy nieces and nephews or the children of friends and neighbors. They not only fill your heart and soothe your weary soul but they also often take you places that you wouldn't ordinarily explore. I wound up thinking, "There's something so therapeutic about watercolors. I might take a class." Sometimes we move so quickly through life that we don't allow ourselves to try new things. Children and grandchildren—your own or other people's—can be a great way to keep you moving in new directions.

FIND ROLE MODELS

Equally important to bolstering self-esteem is finding women who feel good about themselves and their bodies and using them as your role models. Tina Turner is a role model for me. I attended a concert of hers just before she retired at sixty. Although she was dancing next to women half her age, all eyes were glued to her. Why? Because she didn't apologize for her age or her body. She strutted her stuff across the stage, inspiring us all with her energy. Her resiliency shone through.

Another of my role models is Agnes Keleti-Biro, who is the most successful Jewish Olympian ever, and a fireball in her nineties. She survived the Holocaust in wartime Hungary and went on to win ten Olympic medals in gymnastics, five of which were gold. At an October 2001 awards event, where she was inducted into the International Women's Sports Hall of Fame, the audience watched a video of her taped just the summer before. She was filmed doing cartwheels on the beach!

Look around you. What role models do you find inspiring, whether they are athletes, entertainers, business leaders, poets, teachers—or someone who lives just down the street from you. Watch what these role models do. Read their bios, if available, and learn more about their stories. What attributes do they have that you would like to develop yourself? Take one small step toward acquiring those qualities, then another. If you admire an actress, for example, you can take an acting class or rent videos of her plays or movies.

The next time you feel self-conscious about your body, take a cue from your role models—and strut your stuff.

CONFRONT RESISTANCE TO CHANGE

Anxiety about limitations and losses can make us resist change when change is needed. Change doesn't always feel good, even when it's positive, because it also involves loss. That's why it's important to acknowledge and grieve the loss that change brings, and move on.

One woman became aware of the losses of midlife through, of all things, her hair. She had been told all her life that when she turned forty she would have to cut her long dark tresses because long hair would no longer be flattering. "I thought I'd never do that," she said, "but in my forties the texture of my hair and the shape of my face changed. Long hair didn't look so good on me anymore. Since I was always putting it up anyway, I finally got it cut—at age forty-eight. Both I and my husband hated it. It took me two years to find a good haircut."

Hair represents youth, and this woman was fighting the loss of hers. She had to grieve the passing of her youth, and so did her husband. Eventually she began to look through magazines until she found a cut that satisfied her. "I finally realized that I can be an attractive midlife woman with my own signature hairdo and my own personal style. My husband had to grow up and accept this, too."

Another woman, Janice, who is single, sought therapy for depression at age forty-seven. The manager of a weight loss clinic, Janice had lost her passion for life. She spoke of feeling bored, matronly, and sad about her wrinkles and other signs of aging. Her looks had always been her primary source of self-esteem. She had lost her enthusiasm for her work, although she had always read voraciously about weight loss and regularly thought up new strategies.

I asked her to pay attention in upcoming weeks to times when she felt passionate about something, such as getting the chills when hearing someone speak. She reported that while watching TV one night, she heard a young woman candidate on the Republican state ticket and felt inspired by her. We then talked about what she could do next. She proceeded to research the candidate, then decided to volunteer for her campaign. This move led her to meet other volunteers. At fund-raisers she attended, she met other interesting people.

Gradually, her life became quite exciting. She couldn't wait to watch the news to see her candidate. She even got to know the woman and shared her own ideas about the health problem of obesity. She felt passionate about something again and less depressed. Following important campaign issues and putting her time and money into something that interested her helped her feel positive about herself again. Although her body was still important to her, allowing herself to be involved in this cause expanded her horizons. She was respected for her ideas and contributed something to the community that had nothing to do with her looks.

There are many other forms of change in midlife. For example, as a mother, you may have to deal with shifts in your relationship with an adult child. In one of my workshops, a retired librarian spoke of the sadness she felt when her daughter and four-year-old grandson left to move in with the daughter's boyfriend. "I know it's best for them—my daughter needs to have a life—but they brought such joy to the house. I now accept in my fifties that life is full of loss, but I want to enjoy the good stuff, too. I've learned that taking time to grieve my losses helps me to clear them away so I can embrace the pleasures in life."

Her daughter's move had stirred up memories of the loss of her own mother. Fortunately, she realized that she had survived her mother's death and could use that experience as a template for dealing with her daughter's move. She also worked hard to avoid laying a guilt trip on her daughter, as her own mother had done to her. She told her daughter, "I'll miss you, but I know you can do this." This allowed her daughter the opportunity to feel the competency and self-esteem that would come from being able to get out on her own.

To make room for a new vision, you have to grieve that old ways of seeing the world are changing. Part of your sadness may be grieving an old way of being where you may have depended on others to take care of you—or the loss of your dream that a knight in shining armor would always be there. Even changing your role to take better care of yourself involves loss. If people have always told you how wonderful and loving you are because you always put others' needs first, you now have to develop a new identity as someone who knows who she is, knows what she has to do to take care of herself, and is doing it.

REVISIT YOUR VIEW OF THE SEVENTIES

Often our motivation to change and grow is blocked by preconceived notions we have of older women. I see women in my midlife groups freeze in fear at the thought of reaching their seventies. I believe a great deal of this distress about aging has to do with media stereotypes of older women. Although there are many women in their seventies (and older) who are vibrant and alive, we rarely see them in magazines or on TV. It's as if they are invisible. When an elderly woman is pictured, she's usually shown with her grandchildren, rather than in any other role.

Jackie, a participant in one of my groups, changed her opinion of women in their seventies when her mother-in-law was diagnosed with early signs of Alzheimer's. A widow, the mother-in-law always spends a few winter months in Arizona. This time, Jackie accompanied her to get her settled and make sure a nurse's aide was set up to look in on her every day. When Jackie returned home, she reported a surprising experience.

"I had never seen this side of my mother-in-law," she said. "She has lots of friends there, and as soon as we arrived she called them up and said, 'Tomorrow night I'm having a cocktail party. Don't make plans for dinner because I'll have so much food.' We spent the next day buying hors d'oeuvres, vodka, and wine. When the guests arrived (one man and eight women), they were dressed for a ball. The evening, which lasted from 6:30 to 10:30 P.M., was a blast. My mother-in-law was a little forgetful, but I never knew she could be so much freer there than when she is home.

"It also made me feel hopeful about getting older. I always said, 'I don't want to be like my mother-in-law, that single seventy-four-year-old woman who I feel sorry for.' All of a sudden I thought, 'Why am I feeling sorry for her? She has a full life.' "

Another woman in Jackie's group echoed her fears: "I hate the idea of being seventy-five and alone because of my own mother. All she talks about is, 'I met so-and-so and she has cancer, and it's so lonely. None of us have our husbands anymore.' I can't bear that image of myself."

I asked others in the group, "What images do you have of women at seventy-five?"

One participant described her first yoga class with an instructor who is seventy-six years old. "I walked into class and thought, 'Why did I sign up for this? This instructor is too old.' I noticed, however, that the class was full. When we got started, the instructor stretched and moved like someone a quarter her age. And she is this incredibly wise woman. She said things such as, 'I know this is going to hurt a little, but that happens when you're making changes. You're going to find lots of changes in your life when you take yoga.' The two-hour class went by in what seemed like ten minutes. I can't wait to return. Many women repeat her class again and again just to be around her."

Think about becoming a seventy-five-year-old woman in your own mind. Say:

I live in ＿＿＿＿＿＿＿＿ .

I engage in these activities: ＿＿＿＿＿＿＿＿＿＿＿

＿＿＿＿＿＿＿＿＿＿＿＿＿＿＿＿＿＿＿＿＿＿＿＿

＿＿＿＿＿＿＿＿＿＿＿＿＿＿＿＿＿＿＿＿＿＿＿＿

My friends are _____

_____

My feelings about men are _____

_____

_____

Causes that are important to me include _____

_____

_____

_____

What comes out may surprise you. For example, there's no age at which sex has to stop, although it may happen less frequently and there are modifications in activity. People in their seventies and older are often still sexually active, finding sex a source of nourishment and energy.

It is frightening to think of being seventy-five, living without a husband or partner, and stuck with no life. But that scenario doesn't have to be your life. Some women blossom as widows, rediscovering parts of themselves that were submerged in marriage and developing skills they didn't have time for before. The friends of Jackie's mother-in-law went to parties, had a ball at their book club, and generally enjoyed their lives.

At seventy-five, a great-grandmother plays tennis twice a week with a group of men and women who are all younger than she is. She used to play with three men, until their schedule became inconvenient. She also takes a weekly aerobics class. After painting portraits for many years, she now teaches classes in her home and has also taken up sculpture.

French actress Jeanne Moreau, seventy-five, not only continues to appear in films but she's a director as well. In an article in *The New York Times*,[2] she was quoted saying, "To me, life is going up until you are burned by flames. Life is an accomplishment and each moment has a meaning and you must use it." On another occasion, during a television interview, Moreau commented, "I don't mind the wrinkles." Instead, she focused on the importance of curiosity.

We have to be deliberate about noticing such older women, who lead satisfying, enriching lives, and learn from them.

FLAUNT IT

You can be the one at your high school or college class reunion who's vibrant and appealing today—not because you've had a face-lift or lost thirty pounds but because you're alive. Grown-up appeal, sexual and otherwise, is about attitude and energy, strength inside and out, and openness to possibilities. Those traits are ageless and timeless, and others are drawn to them.

Go ahead and break some rules. Question long-held assumptions about what you can and cannot do as a woman during midlife. Don't be like the polar bear, restricting yourself in a cage that no longer exists. Use the ideas and strategies in this book to create a new vision for your body and self—and let your power surge.

10

HELP YOUR DAUGHTER DEVELOP A POSITIVE BODY IMAGE

Complete as the perfect wings of the jay above your head or the pale stars that mark your birth with nothing but pure light. Daughter, I cannot give you anything so complete or perfect or pure. But I can give you something better. Your body . . . and the fierce love of it that no one can take away.

Linda Nemec Foster,
A History of the Body

Listen to virtually any group of teenage girls and the litany of complaints goes on and on: "I have ugly red hair." "I have mousy brown hair." "I'm too tall." "I'm too short." "I'm flat." "My breasts are humongous." "I'm too fat." "I hate my freckles." "I have zits." Research conducted by the American Association of University Women (AAUW)[1] tells us that girls' self-esteem plummets in adolescence. Although boys' self-esteem drops at this time, too, the decline is less dramatic.

One possible explanation for the phenomenon is girls' negative body image, which develops earlier and earlier these days. I've treated girls as young as age nine for eating disorders; research shows that girls' perceptions of their bodies change at around that time. Instead of viewing a round body as healthy and strong, girls begin to see it as fat. That wasn't so fifty years ago, but a lot has changed since then.

Psychologist Mary Pipher, Ph.D., author of *Reviving Ophelia: Saving the Selves of Adolescent Girls,* described those changes at a professional conference I attended in 2001. She spoke of how much more stressful and difficult life has become for teenagers. Community, which used to be a source of security and adult help for youngsters, has faded in our society, due to demographic shifts. Villages are disappearing, and the world of primary relationships—usually composed of close family—is being replaced by the world of secondary relationships. The village is now the electronic community, a poor and sometimes dangerous substitute for the real thing.

Sioux Indians teach that all adults are responsible for all children, said Pipher, yet many parents feel overwhelmed today. No one is there to take over for Mom so that she can rest, because extended family often lives far away. Grandma is no longer next door to help out. Even if she does live nearby, she (along with the neighbors) is likely to be out working herself. And there's nothing in the broader culture that promotes connection between adults and children. In fact, children are often taught to be frightened of adult strangers.

To a large extent, the media have fueled the vacuum. TV, movies, and teen magazines present blatantly sexual content and glorify anorexic stars and sultry, seductive fifteen-year-olds as female idols. In *Reviving Ophelia,* Mary Pipher calls today's sexualized, media-dominated culture "girl poisoning."

Pipher talked, too, of another loss for children: the loss of "ascribed," rather than earned, status in families. In the past, when families lived closer together, a child had status simply by being part of the family, not because she scored well on the SAT. But today ascribed status is largely gone, along with the security it provided for children. Today youngsters have to earn their status and be good at many things.

We see this loss of ascribed status being acted out today in the emphasis on overachievement. Many children are focused on what schools they will get into, rather than on the joy of learning. At six years old, they're in soccer camp to improve their skills, instead of out playing with their friends for the pure pleasure of the game, and feeling good about themselves and the world.

This is the climate in which adolescent girls grow up today, stripped of crucial supports and assaulted by expectations that weaken, rather than strengthen, their sense of self. In response, girls seek acceptance and status, and one way to have status is to look a certain way. In research done at Columbia University, we found an increase in interest in plastic surgery among adolescent girls.[2] Some of the girls even viewed starving or purging themselves, smoking, and plastic surgery as ways to attain a perfect body. Obviously this is a very dangerous development.

For some girls the drive for thinness is fueled right at home by their parents. For the first time in history, young women have been raised by mothers who are critical of their own bodies and who often obsess about the size of their daughters' bodies from the delivery room on.[3] We know from research that mothers who criticize their own bodies criticize their daughters' bodies, and their daughters engage in more extreme dieting techniques.

In short, adolescence, which seems to be a critical time for the development of body image issues, is more turbulent than ever before. How can you help your daughter negotiate it, even if you feel guilty of overvaluing appearance yourself? There is much you can do to help her feel good about her body at this crucial developmental crossroad, and you can begin right now.

KNOW WHAT'S GOING ON DEVELOPMENTALLY

Adolescence is a transition on the way to adulthood. It is the period of physiological and psychological development from onset of puberty to maturity. Today the span from ages ten to thirteen tends to be viewed as early adolescence, a particularly difficult period for girls because it involves not just one single event but a number of major events in a short period of time: the onset of menses, a newly developing body, and changes in self-esteem. The years from fourteen to seventeen are considered middle adolescence; eighteen to the mid-twenties is late adolescence.

Puberty begins when the sex glands receive a signal from the pituitary gland to increase production of estrogen, the female hormone. Estrogen is a good thing. It strengthens bones, acts on the liver to manufacture good cholesterol, and encourages the release of chemicals that elevate mood and boost emotional awareness.

When girls begin to menstruate, weight gain ensues. The effect of the weight on a girl's shape is dramatic: She develops breasts, her hips broaden, and the rest of her body fills out. Skin may break out, and girls feel confusing new emotions.

TALK ABOUT IT

To empower your daughter, tell her what changes to expect and how they are going to affect her body image. Many parents assume that this discussion takes place in school, and sometimes it does. But often the subject is handled in a very technical way. What's missing is the human touch and the sense of connection to a caring adult that you are uniquely able to provide. Your daughter needs to know that what she is going through is perfectly normal, experienced by all girls—and that she is on her way to becoming a woman.

Tell her that she is probably going to grow about ten inches from the onset of puberty to maturation—and put on thirty or forty pounds. At the beginning, estrogen adds weight around the waist. Eleven-, twelve-, and thirteen-year-olds often have big waists, but eventually the weight is redistributed to all areas of the body, especially breasts and hips. This knowledge is essential because girls often worry, "Oh my goodness, I've got a belly like my mother's."

Some girls become so self-conscious of their bodies at this time that they may suddenly refuse to wear a bathing suit anymore or go swimming. If that's your daughter's reaction, let her pick out her clothes and wear cutoffs instead of a bathing suit if she wants to. Her feelings need to be respected.

It's crucial to educate and reassure your daughter because negative body image and eating disorders often develop at this time. Some girls who don't like the way they look start to diet. They think the problem is that they are fat—and that if they reduce, all will be well.

ENCOURAGE PHYSICAL STRENGTH, RATHER THAN THINNESS

Your reaction to your daughter's new body is pivotal. Whatever you do, don't watch what she eats and comment, "Fruit is better for you than a candy bar." Don't make a big deal about her weight or encourage her to diet. Such encouragement has been linked with increased dieting and with bingeing.[4] If your daughter has decided on her own that she wants to lose weight, and you feel it would be helpful, you can, however, support her in healthy eating.

Society tells us to go in there and fix it, but evidence shows that children pushed to diet at a young age get into trouble regulating food intake themselves. "Kids need to learn how to take care of themselves, and they need to be told they're okay. Too many of them grow up in dieting homes that tell them they're not okay," says Sondra Kronberg, M.S., R.D., C.D.N., Nutritional Director of Eating Disorder Associates Treatment and Referral Centers of New York.

One way for your daughter to feel okay is to experience her body as a positive, effective part of her. If she's chubby, teach her to honor how her body functions, not just how it looks, and how strong she can be. Offer many opportunities to try different types of movement that will let her feel her body's responsiveness, develop coordination, and build stamina.

She may not have many choices at school, where physical education programs are frequently slashed to compensate for a menu of computer classes, so you have to do your part. If gymnastics or tennis don't appeal to her, maybe horseback riding, ice-skating, dance, or martial arts will. As she masters her body, she will feel its competence and develop confidence. Physical activities help children develop important life skills, such as discipline, the ability to set and achieve goals, and taking appropriate risks. They can also lead your daughter to feel healthy and energetic, and they help burn calories. Another option is organized team sports, which teach girls to trust their bodies and allow them to express healthy aggression. Over 11 million girls (48 percent) play team sports today, according to *American Demographics* magazine, with soccer being their number one choice. Softball is the runner-up, followed by basketball. Team sports are a great way for girls to learn how to cooperate and compete, which are important skills to develop for the rest of their lives.

THE THREAT OF ANOREXIA AND BULIMIA

For some girls, the focus on weight can lead to bulimia nervosa (binge eating and purging), or anorexia nervosa (self-starvation and severe weight loss), the most lethal of all psychiatric disorders. Today we know that more girls are afflicted with eating disorders than boys are, and girls are becoming increasingly preoccupied with food, developing eating problems at younger ages.

Eating disorders are multidetermined. Research has shown that genetic, psychological, and sociocultural factors play a role in development of anorexia nervosa and bulimia.[5] They are not about what you eat or look like. They're really about how you feel about yourself, and how well you are able to handle feelings, relationships, and issues of competency and control. Some eating disorders begin as an attempt to lose weight and develop into an obsession about control, power, and perfection. A youngster may feel, "If I can't control my parents getting divorced or how my friends treat me, I can at least control what I eat." Some girls use food as a way to soothe or manage their feelings.

How can you recognize signs of anorexia? Commonly, a youngster:

- reduces food intake.
- claims to be fat even if it clearly is not true.
- obsesses about low-calorie, nonfat food choices and often avoids meat.
- denies hunger.
- engages in ritualistic eating tricks, such as dicing meat into tiny pieces and hiding it under the lettuce or potatoes.
- always has an excuse to skip meals.
- tends to be very self-critical.
- gradually becomes isolated. Instead of going out for pizza with the gang after a basketball game, she comes home and gets on the treadmill.

What are red flag signs of bulimia? Commonly a youngster:

- makes excuses to go to the bathroom after eating, or leaves laxative or diuretic wrappers in the trash can.

- eats lots of food but doesn't seem to gain weight. Or she sneaks large amounts of food from the refrigerator.
- is overly concerned with weight and shape.

Although the appearance of one or two symptoms from either list doesn't necessarily indicate a problem, the appearance of several of them together are cause for concern. If you suspect a problem, sit down and talk with your child. Tell her that you're worried that she may have an eating disorder. Then bring her in to see your physician. Consult with the doctor about making an appointment with a therapist. If your child does have an eating disorder, professional help is essential. A team approach is best, including a therapist (psychologist, social worker), a physician, nutritionist, and sometimes a psychiatrist.

BECOME A CONTAINER OF HOPE

Girls can feel hopeless about certain body changes, which is why it's important to tell your daughter that we all come in different shapes and sizes, and that the goal is to respect and care for her body. She needs to do a lot of the things that you're doing for yourself, such as exercise, eating healthy, and resting when tired. Sharing stories about your own experiences at her age is also very helpful to give her perspective and assure her, "I know you're going to get through this."

I remember when my oldest daughter, Kristin, then a sophomore in high school, developed a bad case of acne on her face. Although I took her to a dermatologist who worked with her, she had a tough year. Since I had acne as a teenager myself, I showed her pictures of me at her age. "I remember how awful it was," I told her. "Once I was in a car with a bunch of kids and I made a comment. Someone retorted, 'Who said that—Pimples?' I felt devastated because those words made the acne real. I was hoping that nobody noticed it because I used all kinds of medication, plus makeup to cover it up."

My husband, who had mild acne as a teen himself, used humor. He told her about the time he had a big pimple on one side of his face. He made her laugh because he acted out how he would turn his head and only let people see the other side.

I also gave Kristin some strategies to help her cope with her own feelings and other people's responses to her at this difficult time. I pointed out that the acne was time limited—it would not last forever. "You have it for a certain amount of time and then it's usually gone. You're doing all the right things to prevent scars," I assured her.

I talked about viewing this experience as an opportunity. She'd complain, "Mom, I can't believe that guys who wanted to take me to the junior prom when I was a freshman don't even talk to me now because of the acne." I advised her to use this chance to see how it feels to be rejected or overlooked because of your appearance.

"This is a time to develop other skills," I told her. "When people are blind, they overdevelop other senses. For example, they learn to be great listeners." Kristin is a very pretty girl, and she's very privileged in that way. The most wonderful thing she learned during her acne year was empathy for other girls who are not as fortunate as she is.

I also helped her focus on her strengths and all the ways she could feel good about herself that have nothing to do with her appearance. "What do you do when the world doesn't validate you?" I asked. "How do you validate yourself? You know we all get old, and there's a point when we don't get the same positive feedback about our looks. How can you still feel valuable and move through space in a way that communicates confidence?"

When the acne was at its worst, what worked best for her was a golf clicker, which helps players keep track of their strokes on the course. I bought one at a sports store, told her to keep it with her, and to click it when she did something that she felt good about. She studied for a test and scored well, click. She talked to someone in the hall whom everyone else seemed to ignore, click. She found cool jeans, click. She danced to a song in her room and felt great, click. As she kept track of all the good things she did each day, she became aware of the many ways she felt pride and pleasure in herself. To reinforce her positive feelings, I asked every evening, "How many clicks today?" The clicker helped her through a particularly painful period of her life.

Height may sometimes be another painful issue in adolescence. Tall girls may feel like misfits when they tower over friends. Mothers can help them see their size as a strength that opens doors. Tell a tall daughter to stand straight and proud, rather than slouch and hide. Perhaps steer her to a sport where her size is a great asset, such as basketball. Find role models with whom she can identify. Show her Lisa Leslie, the Women's National Basketball Association (WNBA) star, who is feminine and attractive—and also the toughest player on the court. I once heard Leslie describe how she hated her big feet and her height when she was in middle school. Yet her size made her career. She is a two-time Olympic-gold medalist and she was named Sportswoman of the Year 2001 for the Women's Sports Foundation.

Is your daughter unhappy with her nose? Point to Sarah Jessica Parker and Barbra Streisand. They've turned their big noses into trademarks, and they are glamorous, accomplished, successful stars. Far from perfect tens, they certainly aren't wallflowers. What a wonderful life lesson to teach your child: how to view imperfections as features that enhance you as a unique presence.

MAKE YOUR HOME A HAVEN

If your daughter is overweight, what she hears at home is going to affect how self-conscious she's going to be and whether she overvalues appearance. It's crucial for her to know that you love and accept her. If she's in a family that's interested in how far they can hike rather than who lost the most weight this week— that's going to make a big difference in what she values and notices. Let her be part of a family that says, "Oh, I spoke to Jenny. She's in graduate school and she's actually teaching class," rather than, "Look at Aunt Millie. She gained ten pounds since Thanksgiving." Or, "Look at Kathryn's daughter. I never knew she'd be so big."

Be aware of the hurt caused by critical comments such as, "Your hair never looks right." Or, "You'll never be thin." Some women tell of their chubby granddaughters asking them quite seriously, "Grandma, do you love me even though I'm fat?"

They've responded, "I love you no matter what," but they feel heartbroken for these children who have learned at home that they're not okay. Do not allow teasing about appearance in your home. Taunts from fathers and brothers can be particularly hurtful. In fact, high levels of body dissatisfaction are associated with a history of being teased as a child.

You can also act as a buffer against society. Teasing is rampant in schools today. To help your youngster deal with it, assure her that "It gets better as you get older." Judgments based solely on appearance happen less often after middle school and high school. You can also ask, "What do you think are some ways you can handle teasing?" My daughter Kristin decided that humor was one answer. If somebody called her Pimple Face, she could exaggerate it with, "Don't call me Kristin anymore. Call me Pimple Face." Humor is a great strategy because it takes the power away from the taunter, who often wants you to feel embarrassed.

A funny comeback reframes the situation. It says, "I feel good about myself, and I'm going to have fun with this."

It's also important to raise awareness in the community of how destructive teasing and bullying can be. Often the attitude at school is: "The child has to learn to handle it." But if your daughter comes home and repeatedly reports humiliating incidents, you need to respond even if she's a twelfth-grader. Ask to meet with the teacher, coach, and/or principal. Tell them, "I think it's your job as an adult in this setting to stop this kind of behavior and tell students that it's not acceptable." Punishments such as Saturday detention speak loud and clear. Your support in such situations means so much to your child.

And there's a way to do it so that no one knows where the complaint originated. For example, in one case, some bullying girls in gym class repeatedly grabbed a classmate's purse, throwing it around and refusing to give it back to her. Tremendously upset at being a target, the girl told her mother, who asked me for advice. I told the mother to inform the gym teacher and ask the teacher to tell the class, "I'm aware of the fact that bullying is going on. For example, people are writing on stalls in the bathroom that a certain person is a bitch. Also, girls' purses are being thrown around in the locker room." That way, the teacher picks on two incidents, not just one, making it harder to figure out the identity of the complainant. What if the teacher doesn't know of a second occurrence? He or she can make something up.

It was also important that the teacher make it clear, "There is a zero tolerance policy for bullying behavior. If it happens again and I find out, the girls involved will get detention. The second time it happens, their parents will come in. The third time the students will be suspended. After that they will be expelled."

DEVELOP RITUALS OF TRANSITION

So many transitions occur in adolescence, and it's your job to help your daughter negotiate them. Rituals can be useful tools for introducing her to good feelings about her new body.

For example, is your daughter ready for her first bra? Make shopping for it an event. Take her to the mall and help her try on several styles to get the proper fit. Buy something pretty. This sets a tone that says, "You're entitled to do good things for yourself that make you feel feminine. You deserve them." Top off your excursion with lunch out, just the two of you. You'll both have fun, and the day will become a memory that she can pass on to her daughter someday.

A participant in one of my workshops described her shopping experience with her beloved ten-year-old, who was just sprouting breasts. "I felt so good that I was right on target with her tender feelings about her body. I hardly talked in the store and let her make the decision over what to buy and when to wear it. It's still in her drawer. When I went through this at her age, I only felt embarrassment. I don't remember my mother making time to take my hand and walk me through it."

Girls are affected by how you value womanhood—and menstruation is the introduction to womanhood. One mother honored the arrival of her daughters' periods with a celebration. She prepared a festive dinner, setting the table with a lovely cloth and candles. The message was, "This is an occasion. Something marvelous has happened." She told them, "Women are special. Only women can have babies. Only women can be mothers." She considered it a rite of passage, noting that "You celebrate when someone gets a driver's license. Certainly entering womanhood deserves recognition too."

Another mom named Dale suggested to her husband that he send flowers to their daughter when her first period arrived. He followed through, and wrote on the card, "I'm so proud of you. Welcome to womanhood." Although both parents wanted to take the girl out for a special dinner, she opted for a mother-daughter night. They ate at a restaurant and looked at photos taken of the daughter at her birth. Mom read parts of a journal she had kept when she was pregnant. Entries described her excitement at having a child on the way and even recounted little talks she'd had with her daughter in the womb.

This sharing also helped Dale's daughter adjust to her difficult periods, which involved very heavy flow, plus nausea. Dale mentioned, too, that she'd gotten her period late—in ninth grade— just as her daughter had. This was important information because girls menstruate earlier than they used to. If all of a girl's friends already have their periods, she might feel different and somehow lacking until she catches up. It's comforting for her to know that she isn't the only female to get her period so late.

For positive balance, Dale also shared that her pregnancies were trouble-free. "I always felt fabulous mentally and physically. I just threw up a few times in the beginning. It was incredibly easy," she said.

MENTOR YOUR DAUGHTER

You have much to offer your daughter in other ways. Researchers have found that when they ask adolescent girls who their mentors are, they tend to answer, "My mother." Don't be afraid to see yourself in that role. As women we tend to devalue our knowledge and our impact, but we have so much to teach.

Inside the home, you can teach your daughter to cook and prepare meals or take care of children. Outside the home, talk to her about what you're learning on the job—or on the church committee. Discuss your failures as well as your successes. She can learn from hearing about lessons learned from mistakes and realizing that nobody achieves success without failures along the way.

Too often as parents we just assume that our children know how to manage situations, but they need our guidance, wisdom, and experience. At the end of my daughter's junior year in high school, she came to me and said, "Mom, I want to run for the student body of the whole school next year. I don't care if I'm president or vice president, but I want one of those positions."

We talked and I said, "Well, you have to come up with what you stand for and what you plan to do. You also need to decide who you want to run with." When she started mentioning her friends, I said, "Kristin, you have to realize that you want votes from many different types of kids. Sometimes it's better to run with somebody who has the same agenda as you do, but who hangs out with a different group and will pull in votes from other students." She wound up running with a boy who wanted to be president, which was okay with her. They both had the same general ideas, but they came from different crowds. They made a great team—and they won the election.

HELP HER SET GOALS

Another way to coach your daughter is to help her set productive goals and figure out how to reach them. Many young girls set their goals around a model, or a TV or movie star. They may even take on a celebrity's identity. They'll come in and say, "I was reading about so-and-so. She drinks this kind of coffee, reads this kind of book, and is on this kind of diet. I'm reading the same book; I drink the same coffee; and I'm on the same one-thousand-calorie-a-day diet that she's on."

We need to help girls make it a goal to develop their own identities, and we need to help them make decisions today that will affect them later. Your daughter might lose weight on a thousand-calorie diet in the short term, but it's not a long-term solution. Talk to her about being more than just a body. Remind her that she is a complete person with talents, abilities, and unique traits. Help her to set her own standards of appearance for herself. Developing healthy self-esteem requires the ability to create a personal vision for oneself. If teenagers do not develop a vision, they will lack a sense of direction and meaning in their lives and will be easily swayed by others.

Teens also need help to realistically achieve goals. Ask a girl to identify her dreams, and she'll often say, "I want to be a pediatrician," or "I want to be rich and not worry about money." Because those are such general goals, however, there are no steps to achieve them. Youngsters get stuck and don't make any progress. To move toward the dream, they need to get specific. Help your daughter by asking the right questions, such as, "Well, what does being rich mean to you? What kind of work would you do to get rich?" She might meet with the school guidance counselor to find out the pay scales for various jobs. Then she might come back and report, "There are six different jobs that pay very well." You can then continue, "Well, what are your talents, skills, and interests? Which job seems to fit you?"

What if your daughter aspires to be a singer in a rock band? Be realistic. You might say, "It's tough to make it in a rock band, but some people succeed. Let's see what you have to do, such as take music lessons." When she discovers all the practice, discipline, and rejection involved in such a career, she may decide it isn't for her after all. You can also mention that some people decide to make a living in a more stable career, yet indulge their passion by singing with a band on weekends.

If your daughter insists on pursuing a career as a singer in a rock band regardless, then get behind her and support her. I know someone whose daughter wanted to be an actress. After graduation from college, she worked in small regional theaters, then went to New York City. But she tired of making no money. She was good, but not good enough. So she got professional career counseling to help her move away from acting into a profession. However, she never regretted pursuing her dream, and she never forgot her mother's support.

THE IMPORTANCE OF DOWNTIME

There's a myth that teenagers don't want to be with their parents. The reality is that they do want to spend some time with us. And they need us more than ever to help them interpret the world because they have access to so much information on sex, drugs, and other issues at younger and younger ages, when they are not equipped to handle them. They need adult advice and guidance about the messages they are receiving. It can seem impossible to find an extra minute, but downtime with your daughter is essential to get closer and stay in touch with what is going on in her life.

Downtime together can be as simple as sharing tasks such as working on the lawn, doing the laundry, or tending to an errand. The two of you might go to the supermarket together, then stop for ice cream or some great-tasting coffee, or shop for sneakers. Sharing activities is vital because teenagers tend to talk to you about important issues when they're doing other things and not making eye contact with you. It may be 10:30 P.M. and you're both exhausted, but you can see it as a quiet time to relax together. Sit in a chair or lie down on the bed in her room, and talk about the day. It's at these quiet times that she is likely to open up about what's on her mind, such as feeling fat or unpopular. Many teenage girls also talk when driving in the car with you. It's often easier for them to share when they're not looking directly at you.

Be quiet and listen to her. If she mentions a problem, don't rob her of the opportunity to solve it herself. Don't immediately jump in to make suggestions, offering advice or solutions. Give her time to express her feelings and describe the details. When you listen, you enable her to listen to herself and begin to do creative problem solving.

This can also be a time when you reflect back her feelings about difficult situations. Called mirroring, this exercise teaches her a language to describe what she was feeling about an experience, instead of just saying, "It was terrible," and leaving it at that.

For example, my younger daughter, Jennifer, who is passionate about dance, attends classes twice a week. However, a part of me wanted her to choose soccer to broaden her interests and meet a whole new group of friends. I asked her, "Do you want to sign up for a sport? You're good at soccer." But she wasn't interested, preferring to stick to dance. I had to accept that, mirror who she is, and tell her, "You're right. This is what you love—to dance."

The fact was, soccer was really *my* need, not hers. I had to stop pushing my agenda and make sure I got excited about *hers*. I validated her with, "Tell me about dance tonight. Show me the steps for the recital."

Such words mirror her, confirming, "Yes, dance is important to you. And because it's important to you, I will support you."

Youngsters who don't know what feelings are, or how to label them, are at risk for trouble. Because they don't know what to do with feelings such as anger or sadness, they may turn to actions such as overeating, drinking, or worse because these actions enable them to escape the pain. When I took a national sample of adolescent girls in 2001, sponsored by an unrestricted educational grant from Secret antiperspirant, I found that 26 percent of girls reported that they burned or cut themselves on purpose. They're actually experiencing mental pain and don't know how to regulate it. They mutilate themselves as a way to switch focus from emotional pain to physical pain, which they feel they can control because they do the cutting or burning. Fifty years ago, only a few girls engaged in such behavior.

For example, perhaps your daughter's close friend is moving far away. Other girls have planned a big going-away party and haven't invited your daughter. She tells you, "I don't even want to go because I know how mean they can be to people, but it feels bad that I'm left out." You can help her enormously by mirroring her painful feelings with something like, "It sounds like you're really disappointed, and even though you don't care to be with these girls, you would like to celebrate your friend. And I wonder if anything else makes you feel bad—like losing a good friend."

Reflecting back validates her feelings. It allows her to discuss the hurt of being left out and admit, "Yeah, you'd think they'd invite me. It hurts when you're not included in a going-away party for someone you like. I'll miss Heather so much."

It's important to help girls talk about feelings and experience competency in the world so they don't have to use an eating disorder or other destructive behavior to exercise some control. These kinds of conversations can only take place, however, when you're both totally relaxed. Everybody is so busy. Kids often go in different directions. One has soccer practice, another has to go to the library or glee club. Yet just hanging out is an activity to cherish. When I was growing up, I remember that Friday night was special. On Friday night, my mother always made homemade pizza. She and my father would have a glass of wine after dinner and talk. Then they'd put Engelbert Humperdinck on the record player and they'd dance. The message was, "This is the end of the workweek, and it's time to have fun together."

What I love about the memory is the fact that I was one of six kids, and everyone was in the house, but there was no pressure. I might go and play in my room a little, then come out and join a conversation with my sister. Or I'd watch TV for a while with my brothers, or I'd just love to watch my parents dancing. Sometimes we children would dance. There was something about having that time together that gave me a deep sense of security.

My husband and I sometimes spend Friday nights that way now to set it apart from the rest of the week. My two older children may be out, but my little ones invite buddies over. We might go down to the basement to play pool, then we come back up to the living room. My husband and I have a glass of wine, and the kids sit and talk to us.

You can start your own designated family downtime, beginning with having dinner together at least three times a week. Sitting down together at a table and sharing food and conversation at the end of the day can be healing for everyone. And there is a bonus—mealtime eating discourages grazing and binge eating.

Include physical activity in your downtime, too. Go biking together and take walks. I remember a family vacation in Florida when my daughter Kristin and I walked every morning on the beach. She called it "the mother-daughter walk," and each day she voiced her anxieties about which colleges might accept her. Although her applications were all in, as a typical senior she worried, "I'm not going to get in anywhere."

I had nothing too profound to say, but I listened and was a container of hope for her. "Wherever you wind up, you're going to make something happen," I assured her. When we got back home, she asked to continue our mother-daughter walks for a few days until her school vacation was over. She needed that downtime to share.

Beware, however, of making dieting a bonding experience between you as you share cottage cheese, diet tips, and recipes. As one patient described it, "My mother and I had a secret society that neither my father nor brother could penetrate." Dieting can become a way to draw closer to others. However, the goal is to bond with your daughter in healthier, more interesting and exciting ways.

DEVELOPING A MORE MATURE CONNECTION

A major task of adolescence involves forming an identity that is separate from parents. The goal is to maintain closeness but develop a different, more adult relationship between you. To develop a firm sense of self, your child has to figure out her own beliefs, values, and dreams. And part of your job is to accept that they will be different from yours in some ways.

Allow your daughter to be herself, rather than a reflection of you. You may have big plans for her to become a CEO, but she may have no interest in business school. Although we all have hopes for our children, they have their own talents and dreams that must be honored. Keep your expectations in line with your child's individual nature. The more realistic you can be, the more you can help her, as well as yourself.

One of the greatest gifts you can give her is to look into her eyes, see who she really is, and encourage her to fulfill her potential. Parents who are able to accept their children as they are, and are able to feel excited about it, raise kids who do well. Why? Because teens who feel that they are seen and understood by their parents for who they really are, are able to be authentic. They don't have to hide parts of themselves because they fear rejection. They internalize your acceptance of all that they are, and can accept and feel good about themselves. This is the cornerstone of healthy self-esteem.

Conversely, children are set up for frustration and potential trouble when they hear, "You may not make it in art, so I'm going to push you into these other classes instead. You're going to need to make a lot of money." Youngsters who don't use their gifts feel bad about themselves and don't do as well as other children.

I see mothers all the time who want their daughters to do what they themselves didn't do. The message is, "I never went to Harvard, but I want you to go." Or, "I never had a career but I want you to have one." In this age of the super child, many parents use their children to climb the ladder of success themselves. For example, some parents in large cities train their children for kindergarten interviews. Since five-year-olds don't care which school they attend, the child's welfare is obviously not the issue. See your child as someone unique and separate, not as a narcissistic extension of yourself. Only then can she flourish.

ARE YOU DISTORTING THE WAY YOU SEE YOUR DAUGHTER?

I sometimes suggest this exercise to mothers who see their daughters as an extension of themselves. Try it yourself. Answer the questions below, together with your own daughter, if possible. Whatever age your daughter is, pretend that you are back at that age yourself. Then remember what life was like for you, and answer accordingly. Fill in the school you attended, your favorite subject, etc.

	Daughter	Mother
1. What school do you go to?		
2. Who is your favorite teacher?		
3. What is your favorite subject?		
4. What do you do after school?		
5. Who are your best friends? Why?		
6. What is the most important event that happened this year?		
7. What are your passionate interests?		
8. What are your dreams?		

As a mother answers the questions herself, she might say, "My dream was to be the prom queen."

I'll ask, "What was it like when you weren't?" The daughter then listens to her mother's answer and can empathize with her disappointment. I'll also inquire, "Do you think your experience affects what you want from your daughter? How? Do you want her to be thin so that she can be the prom queen that you weren't?"

Ask yourself these same questions. It's a way to share and get a discussion going between you and your daughter. You can see ways that you're both the same, ways that you're different, and whether you are distorting how you see your daughter.

Girls whose preferences have been valued by parents are more able to identify what they want, evaluate their accomplishments, and rely more on themselves for direction than looking for approval from others. In contrast, those whose preferences have never been supported develop a very fragile sense of self.

In a common scenario, a mother wants her daughter to shine in a sport, such as tennis. It is the mother's need, not the daughter's. The daughter is actually drawn to the arts. Nevertheless she devotes herself to tennis lessons and practice—and develops a false sense of self. She loses touch with who she is and what she wants. The mother trains her as if she's going to the Olympics, and the girl winds up bingeing at the candy machine. She develops a problem listening to all internal cues, including signals that she is hungry or full. She doesn't know what she wants because her own preferences have never been supported.

A girl who gives up her authentic self feels constant self-doubt and always second-guesses or suppresses her opinions. She looks for attention outside of herself to figure out what she's feeling.

Girls are led to feel that they can compete in only one arena— with other females to look their best, be the most popular with guys, and go to the top camp. This competition affects body image because many girls constantly compare themselves to other girls. If someone is prettier, it can ruin their whole day. Often they judge themselves harshly and negatively, and feel hopeless. It's important to validate them by mirroring emotional strength and intellectual ability, as well as physical attractiveness, because if this attitude continues over time, they are at risk for eating disorders, depression, addiction, and worse.

Mothers also need to resist pushing their own needs in respect to their daughters' appearance. Mothers who were fat themselves as children often want their daughters to be the beautiful, popular girls that they never were.

Years ago, after I was interviewed for an article in *American Health* magazine, I received letters such as this:

> Dear Dr. Cooke,
> I've given up on my body, but I'm concerned about my daughter's. I know this isn't right, but I'm so relieved that she is thin. I don't know if I could ever accept her if she was fat. I love when she doesn't eat all the food on her plate and that when she skips meals, she doesn't seem to care. I love when she's all dressed up and people tell me how cute she is. I brought her up on diet bread and light margarine, and she has such good habits. Isn't that what you should be telling people to do? It's our only hope.

The trouble is, girls in such situations feel enormous pressure to be thin. In rebellion, many overeat.

It may also be hard to accept a chubby child if you were brought up in a family where everyone was expected to be slim and attractive, and outsiders who were not were criticized unmercifully. If you feel mortified that your child is fat, you need to talk about your feelings with someone—your husband, a friend, a therapist. It's important to face and deal with feelings of shame and helplessness so that you can behave like an adult and be compassionate and helpful to your child.

HELP IDENTIFY VALUES

Your daughter has to answer the question, "Who am I?" which isn't easy today. Because we are such a body-and appearance-oriented culture, "Who am I?" is often replaced with "What should I look like?" Or, "What image do I want to project?"

To help girls clarify their personal values and know what they stand for, I often ask them to draw a circle in the center of a sheet of paper, and list in the circle the values that are important to them, such as honesty, sexual orientation, virginity, education, open-mindedness, tolerance, or the environment. I tell them to look at each one and think, "If I did not have this value, would I still be me—or would I be another person?" If the answer is, "I would still be me," the value is crossed out and moved to a list outside the circle. What's left inside are their nonnegotiable values, which vary from person to person. For one person, tolerance may be a value that is held to be politically correct; for another it can be a passionate commitment.

You can ask your own daughter to try the exercise, to clarify which are her core values and which are less important and negotiable. Try the exercise along with her to get in touch with your own values. Then you can compare your results. As a mother you need to be able to accept that your daughter has different likes and dislikes and feels different about certain issues, such as politics. Only then can you develop a relationship based on mutual trust and respect.

Knowing what she stands for will also help your daughter set boundaries and maintain the integrity of who she is. Without boundaries, it becomes too easy to put others' needs before her own. She can find herself doing things she doesn't want to, such as taking drugs, having sex when she's not ready, or developing an eating disorder.

When your daughter understands her values, she's likelier to know when her boundaries are being violated and be able to say no when she feels uncomfortable or that something is not right. Teach her to listen to signals that tell her an action will betray the integrity of her true self. Teach her that it's okay to say no, state her needs, respect herself, and expect to be respected by others—that she has a right to privacy and a right to change her mind. Girls often tell me that they sit at a lunch table and someone will say, "My parents are out of town this weekend. I want you all to sleep over and we'll have a party. Just tell your parents my folks are going to be in town." Everyone responds, "Oh it will be fun, and we'll invite these guys." They all get into it, and there is lots of peer pressure to join in.

As the day goes by, however, girls begin to think, "It sounds like fun, except everybody will probably get drunk, including my boyfriend. He'll probably get pushy sexually. I don't want to be in that situation, but I'll look like a loser if I say I'm not coming."

It's important to redefine for that girl that she is not being a loser. She is someone who is thoughtful and clear about what she wants to do and not do, and there is strength in saying, "Listen, I appreciate your asking me, but I'm not going to be able to do that. Let's do something next week after school." That's setting a boundary.

EXPECT FLAK

In the course of developing her own unique identity, your daughter may put you down. It's important that you are clear with your daughter that it's not okay to be rude, but it's okay to have different opinions. Try not to take it personally. Girls are usually in an intense relationship with their mothers. Putting you down is a way of declaring, "I'm not like you, I'm my own person." One of the things girls do at this time is idealize other moms and give you a hard time. You'll be told that a friend's mother works, and that's more admirable than staying home as you do, or vice versa. You'll hear, "I want you to be like her. She's a good mother; you're a bad mother." Or, "She lets her daughter have green hair." Often the closer you are, the more angry she may get as she attempts to be separate from you.

I remember a girl who came up to talk to me after a teen workshop. "My mother is really a good mother, not like some of the mothers girls talked about today," she said. "But why am I so angry at her? I'm mad because she leaves the lights on in the basement. I'm mad that she leaves things in the refrigerator too long and then we have to eat them."

I suggested that she did have a great mother and didn't have much to be mad about, so she picked on little things because she had to separate. I told her, "Maybe the way to have a different relationship with her is to think about what your opinions and views are and what you want out of life. You'll probably find that some are similar to your mom's and some are different. Maybe that can be a way to be separate so that you don't have to pick on her for little things."

Only with separation is it possible for your daughter to return to a normal relationship with you. During separation, she comes to terms with you, accepting you with all your imperfections, which allows her to do that with herself. It's a big step.

During the separation process, a daughter may not even believe what she is saying. She may just say it to get a reaction and show she is standing on her own. She may declare, "I believe in women's rights," when she knows that you are not a feminist. Or she may make some other provocative statement if she knows that you are a feminist.

In such cases, the best response is, "Tell me about that. Tell me more." And it's also okay to respond, "Gee, I see it totally different from you, but I want to hear more about your thoughts on this issue."

While your daughter is finding her identity, you have to be the adult and say to yourself, "This is a clumsy time right now. She's trying to establish her identity and a way to be close, and I have to stay calm. When she asks, 'Why do you always have to leave the lights on? Nobody else's mother does that,' I have to understand enough about the development of teenage girls to know that I don't have to turn that into a major fight. I'll pick my battles."

BE A ROLE MODEL FOR GOOD EATING HABITS

One of the ways girls develop body image is through identification with the same-sex parent. Think about the messages your attitudes and behaviors toward your own body send your daughter. She incorporates and identifies with your body image as part of her body image. Research suggests that if you diet and binge, you may increase the risk of obesity in your children through role modeling of unhealthy eating behaviors.[6] But you can positively influence your daughter's self-image, body image, and eating attitudes even if you don't feel positive about yourself in these areas by modeling a new, healthy attitude toward your own body. You've learned how to determine a realistic weight and shape for yourself. Put time aside to exercise and eat healthy. Relax your body each day. Take care of it, and that doesn't just mean exercise. It means getting a pap smear and a mammogram. When children see you taking care of yourself, they assume that it is normal behavior.

Show her good eating habits by providing meals that are wholesome and move away from fast foods. The latter are part of the reason for the dramatic rise in childhood obesity, which puts youngsters at risk for diabetes, heart disease, and many other health problems. An estimated 15 percent of children and adolescents ages six to nineteen are overweight now, more than twice the number in the early 1970s, according to results of the 1999–2000 National Health and Nutrition Examination Survey. Think about how you and your daughter can share downtime together cooking a meal.

Girls at increasingly younger ages worry about the shape and weight of their bodies. Many girls feel that they should diet and be really careful about eating. Often if they do that, they'll crave high-fat foods, which can lead to bingeing. They will start to lose weight, then gain it in a destructive cycle. The reality is unless you stay on a strict diet all your life you can't maintain the loss.

To prevent or stop the cycle, encourage your daughter to do the following:

- *Eat all meals, especially breakfast.* Meal skipping is one of the reasons for the increase in adolescent girls' weight. When they try to cut calories that way they actually slow down their metabolism and disrupt the body's natural calorie-burning system. Eating nutritionally adequate foods at regular intervals helps minimize cravings.

- *Pay attention to her body's signals and respond to them.* Girls often say to me, "I don't know when I'm full because I'm always trying not to eat too much." I ask them to start a food journal to keep track of how hungry and full they are before and after they eat. Then I tell them to ask, "How hungry am I?" and rate themselves on a scale of one to ten, with one standing for famished, and ten for stuffed or so full it hurts.

- *View food as energy.* Your daughter is at a time of life when she needs a lot of energy. It's important to keep her body fueled to handle her busy schedule. But she must be aware of the type of fuel she eats. Soda consumption is a big factor in kids' obesity, as are fast-food meals with portions that have become super-sized and tend to be high in both fat and calories.

- *Avoid nibbling when reading, watching TV, or doing homework.* If your daughter needs snacks during the day to meet her calorie and nutrient needs, she can have snacks. However, because it's easier to overeat when you're not paying attention to what you're eating, advise her to stop all other activities when snacking and be mindful of her food.

- *Stop focusing on nonfat foods.* "The increase in kids' obesity is due to the move to eliminate (decrease) fat, while increasing (substituting) refined carbohydrates in diets since 1970," says nutritionist Sondra Kronberg. Your daughter needs to eat what her body tells her it needs, and that includes fat. Try to maintain a balance of nutritious foods in her diet, along with occasional less-healthy snacks. Remember, she can gain weight if she overeats nonfat foods. I know a teenager who nibbles licorice all day, which is nonfat. But she continually adds pounds, because the calories add up.

- *Learn more ways to enjoy food.* Suggest that your daughter go to the grocery store and pick some foods she's never tried before, such as a different kind of fruit, vegetable, pasta, or cereal. Encourage her to try making a few recipes on her own.

- *Find other ways to fill herself up and figure out what satisfies her.* If she's bored, food is not the answer. Your daughter needs to focus on more productive things in her life that make her feel good, such as school, extracurricular activities, and friends.

- ***Choose supportive friends and avoid those who aren't.***
  We know from research that females grow when they are in healthy relationships with one another. In fact, when girls are isolated and disconnected from others, they begin to develop symptoms of depression, anxiety, and other conditions. But they need to know the difference between positive and negative relationships. Teach your daughter that in healthy relationships, friends support, affirm, and like her. They don't put her down, encourage her to engage in destructive behaviors such as shoplifting or drinking, or behave disloyally to her.

Take care of your child. Tell her, "We love you. We care about you. We want to support you in staying healthy and strong." Says nutritionist Sondra Kronberg, "Your child needs one person in the world who thinks the moon and stars rise on her—and that person is usually you."

You can fulfill your potential as a parent, and as a woman, by building a strong body, mind, and spirit. Remember that the body is the house you live in. Take time to choose a realistic weight goal for yourself, and eat and live in a mindful way. Talk positively about your body and compliment other women around you about theirs. Too often, mothers and daughters and other women get together, complain about how they look, and trade weight-loss strategies, which only fuels bad feelings about themselves. But you can change that experience into something positive and powerful, a ritual wherein women validate each other and share stories about their passions and dreams. Imagine how this will affect you and the young women around you.

Let's be courageous and leave a legacy for young women to follow.

Let's develop our own ideal of beauty, and stop looking outward to media messages and to fashion. Instead, let's look within to find the best way to care for our bodies and express who we are. It's time to be more, not less, in midlife, to pay more attention to our health and goals, and teach others how to treat our bodies.

The next phase of the women's movement can begin right now, as we speak our wisdom and share our ideas. Our generation can launch a whole new positive body image movement for women. Let it start with you.

ENDNOTES

Introduction

1. M. A. Gupta, "Concerns About Aging and a Drive for Thinness: A Factor in the Biopsychosocial Model of Eating Disorders," *International Journal of Eating Disorders,* 18 (1995):351–357.
2. K. J. Zerbe, "Eating Disorders in Middle and Late Life, a Neglected Problem," *Primary Psychiatry,* 10, 6 (2003):80–82.
3. Sara Wilcox, "Age and Gender in Relation to Body Attitudes," *Psychology of Women Quarterly* (Cambridge University Press) 21 (1997):549–565.
4. D. M. Lewis and F. M. Cachelin, "Body Image, Body Dissatisfaction, and Eating Attitudes in Midlife and Elderly Women," *Eating Disorders, The Journal of Treatment and Prevention* 9 (2001):29–39.
5. P. A. J. Kay, "Clinical Aspects of Geriatric Eating Disorders," N. H. Field and B. Domangue (eds.), *Eating Disorders Throughout the Life Span* (Praeger) (New York):139–146.
6. Madhulika A. Gupta and Nicholas J. Schork, "Aging Related Concerns and Body Image: Possible Future Implications for Eating Disorders," *International Journal of Eating Disorders* 14, (1993) no. 4:11.
7. Sara Wilcox, "Age and Gender in Relation to Body Attitudes," *Psychology of Women Quarterly* (Cambridge University Press) 21 (1997):549–565.

Chapter 2

1. R. H. Striegel-Moore and A. Kearney-Cooke, "Exploring Parents' Attitudes and Behaviors about Their Children's Physical Appearance," *International Journal of Eating Disorders* 15 (1994):377–385.
2. F. C. MacGregor et al., *Facial Deformities and Plastic Surgery* (Springfield, IL: Thomas, 1953).
3. R. Levinson, B. Powell, and L. C. Steelman, "Social Location, Significant Others and Body Image among Adolescents," *Social Psychology Quarterly* 49 (1986):330–337.
4. A. Kearney-Cooke, and D. M. Ackard, "The Effects of Sexual Abuse on Body

Image, Self-image, and Sexual Activity of Women," *The Journal of Gender-Specific Medicine* 3[6] (2000):54–60.

5. S. C. Wooley and O. W. Wooley, "Feeling Fat in a Thin Society," *Glamour,* February 1984, 198–202.

6. American Psychiatric Association, *The Diagnostic and Statistical Manual for Mental Disorders,* 4th ed. (Washington, D.C.:American Psychiatric Association, 1994).

7. C. V. Wiseman, J. J. Gray, J. E. Mosimann, and A. H. Ahrens, "Cultural Expectations of Thinness in Women: An Update," *International Journal of Eating Disorders* 11 (1) (1990):85–89.

8. A. Allaz et al., "Body Weight Preoccupation in Middle-age and Aging Women: A General Population Survey," *International Journal of Eating Disorders* 23 (1998):287–294.

Chapter 3

1. G. A. Bray, "The Inheritance of Corpulence," in *Weight Regulatory System: Normal and Disturbed Mechanisms,* eds. L. A. Cioffi, W. P. T. James, and T. B. Vanitallie (New York. Raven Press, 1981), 185–195.

2. J. Rotter, "Generalized Expectancies for Internal Versus External Reinforcement," *Psychological Monographs,* 80 (1966):1–69.

Chapter 5

1. American College Sports Medicine, *Resource Manual for Guidelines for Exercise Testing and Prescription,* 2nd ed. (Philadelphia: Lea & Febiger 1993).

2. "Game for Anything: The Strength of Women in Sports," *ABC's Wide World of Sports,* 12/9/2000.

Chapter 6

1. S. Wolin and S. Wolin, *The Resilient Self* (New York: Villard Books, 1993).

Chapter 8

1. Richard Rothstein, "Achievers and Delinquents Via Melting Pot Recipe," *New York Times,* 24 April 2002, Lessons section.

2. F. M. Cachelin, R. H. Striegel-Moore, and K. A. Elder, "Realistic Weight Perception and Body Size Assessments in a Racially Diverse Community Sample of Dieters," *Obesity Research* 6 (1998):62–68.

Chapter 9

1. D. W. Winnicott, *Maturational Processes and the Facilitating Environment* (New York: International Universities Press, 1965).
2. *The New York Times,* 13 January 2001. "Like Acting and Loving, Honor Suits Jeanne Moreau."

Chapter 10

1. American Association of University Women, *How Schools Shortchange Girls.* (New York: Marlowe, 1995).
2. A. Kearney-Cooke, M. Lagota, and D. Ackard, "Cosmetic Surgery among Female Youth: Associations with Family and Peer Relationships, Self-esteem, Body Image, and Risk Behaviors" (paper presented at the International Academy of Eating Disorders meeting, Vancouver, BC, May 19, 2001).
3. S. C. Wooley and A. M. Kearney-Cooke, "Intensive Treatment of Bulimia and Body Image Disturbance," in *Physiology, Psychology and the Treatment of Eating Disorders,* eds. K. D. Brownell and J. P. Foreyt (New York: Basic Books, 1986), 477–501.
4. R. Levinson, B. Powell, and L. C. Steelman, "Social Location, Significant Others and Body Image among Adolescents," *Social Psychology Quarterly,* 49 (1986):330–337.
5. C. M. Bulik, P. F. Sullivan, T. E. Weltzin, and W. H. Kaye, "Temperament in Eating Disorders," *International Journal of Eating Disorders* 17 (1995):251–261.
6. M. Y Hood, L. L. Moore, A. Sundaraan-Ramamurti, M. Singer, L. A. Cupples, and R. C. Ellison, "Parental Eating Attitudes and the Development of Obesity in Children: The Framingham Children's Study," *International Journal of Obesity* 24:(2000) 1319–1325.

Index